Emerging Models for Global Health in Radiation Oncology

Emerging Models for Global Health in Radiation Oncology

Wilfred Ngwa
Dana Farber/Harvard Cancer Center and University of Massachusetts, Lowell, MA, USA

Twalib Ngoma
Muhimbili University of Health and Allied Sciences, Tanzania

IOP Publishing, Bristol, UK

ISBN 978-0-7503-1224-0 (ebook)
ISBN 978-0-7503-1225-7 (print)
ISBN 978-0-7503-1226-4 (mobi)

DOI 10.1088/978-0-7503-1224-0

Version: 20160301

IOP Expanding Physics
ISSN 2053-2563 (online)
ISSN 2054-7315 (print)

British Library Cataloguing-in-Publication Data: A catalogue record for this book is available from the British Library.

Published by IOP Publishing, wholly owned by The Institute of Physics, London

IOP Publishing, Temple Circus, Temple Way, Bristol, BS1 6HG, UK

US Office: IOP Publishing, Inc., 190 North Independence Mall West, Suite 601, Philadelphia, PA 19106, USA

We have a dream that one day cancer will be eradicated and that people of all socio-economic, racial, religious and cultural backgrounds will have access to quality treatment. We dedicate this book to anyone dealing with cancer, and especially to those in low and middle income countries in Asia, Africa, Latin America, eastern Europe and elsewhere who have little or no access to cancer treatment and radiotherapy.

W Ngwa and T Ngoma

Contents

Preface

Global health is an emerging multisectoral field, which brings together the best of science, medicine and humanity. It is a field where we recognize that in today's world *global health is local health and local health is global health*, a field where everyone can participate, linking the healthcare industry, economics, governance and foreign policy, the diaspora, and development and humanitarian aid. With cancer costing millions of lives and trillions of US dollars across the world each year, people are increasingly coming together across institutions, cultures, countries and continents to work with a greater sense of purpose and urgency to stop this growing scourge. This book recognizes the need for a resource that can serve as a useful reference for the emerging field of global health in radiation oncology, as we reach across disciplines at all levels (from the individual/volunteer level to the supranational level) in transformative collaborations to close the cancer divide, save lives and advance globally beneficial socio-economic development.

We have a dream that one day cancer will be eradicated and that people of all socio-economic, racial, religious and cultural backgrounds will have access to quality treatment and cures. The sample stories that follow have inspired this dream at the individual level and motivated greater collaborative global health action towards the elimination of global cancer disparities.

***

Patient (in low income country)
I am 26 years old and recently I was diagnosed with urinary tract infection (UTI). After the diagnosis the doctor decided to order further tests which concluded that I had a tumor on my right kidney. It was recommended that I undergo surgery immediately to prevent possible metastasis if the tumor turned out to be malignant.

I shared the news with my family, but because my mother had just passed, my uncle assumed the responsibility of the elder in the family and decided to see the doctor for clarification. Unfortunately the doctor was very unhappy that I sent someone to question him.

On 20 July 2014, just about two weeks from my diagnosis, I underwent surgical removal of my right kidney (right radical nephrectomy). Since then, I have not been okay; my stomach has swollen, I have no appetite and sometimes I experience vomiting of a yellow substance.

The doctor told me everything was going to be okay after the surgery, but I am not sure exactly what he found because he did not give me any report. I asked him if he saw the tumor and if it is cancerous, but he said the kidney has been disposed of. So I am requesting if you can find any help for my condition.

Intervention (a Good Samaritan residing in the USA)
We could try to advocate for you but you need to get your report, at least know the actual diagnosis so we can try to get a second opinion.

Patient
It is almost two months now since I requested the report from the doctor. I reported to him that I have not been feeling well and he asked me to meet him but not at the hospital, he suggested to meet him at a convenient store or sometimes at a bus stop [...] Finally I have a report [...] but some of the symptoms written I have never really experienced.

"To whom it may concern—re: XXX, *76* yrs, female, hosp. reg. no. XXX"
The above named underwent right radical nephrectomy in July 2014. Intra-operative findings were a tumor within Gerota's fascia but not beyond and solitary para-aortic lymphnode enlargement on the right side. Histology revealed the papillary renal cell carcinoma lymphnode was free of malignancy. She recently presented with fever, weight loss and right hypochondrial pain. Abdominal ultrasound revealed hepatic tumor and FNAC revealed cellular features of malignancy. The CT scan revealed a tumor involving the right hepatic lobe of the liver and enhancing with contrast suggested liver metastasis. The chest x-ray revealed tenting of the right hemidiaphragm and elevated right hemidiaphragm. Serum creatinine is 92 umol/l. Liver function tests are normal, Hb 11.1 g/dl, WBC and RBCC are normal; PLT 576 is high. Alpha fetoprotein is normal, 0.50 IU/ml, PT is 12.5 which is slightly elevated. PTT is normal 30.1, INR is 1.1 normal. We have an impression of metastatic RCC post nephrectomy. Kindly assist for possible targeted therapy or immunotherapy. Dr XXX, Consultant Urological Surgeon.

Intervention
Please go to facility B, take your report there and ask them to run all necessary tests to find out the current/actual problem and make sure you share all the symptoms and history before your surgery so you can get a second opinion.

Patient
Update: facility B reviewed the report from facility A and said that there is nothing they can do for me. I asked them for a referral to India as they send other patients, but they said at this point India will not be able to do anything [...] I am not feeling well sometimes I am in so much pain sometimes I feel very weak. I have asked my family not to talk about my condition, so we do not talk about it because there is nothing we can do. All I ask God is to wake up and find that I am healed.

Intervention
Send me a copy of your report and please allow me to share with doctors in the field so we get the best advice. Report and images were shared with an oncologist in a developed country:

1. error noted on age;
2. patient denied some of the reported symptoms prior to the surgery;
3. inconclusive, advocate for patient to be reviewed in facility B with more tests or any other facility possible.

Another doctor within the continent has agreed to see the patient, unfortunately we could not raise enough funds for travel and patient care costs.

November 2015

We managed to get someone who will meet the patient locally at facility B and make it possible for facility B to accept the patient and reevaluate the patient irrespective of the report from facility A.

Patient advised to make a list of all present physical concerns/ history and report to the doctor in facility B.

Patient

I went to facility B and I met with the person you referred me to, he talked to the doctor and I was assigned a doctor right away. They ordered some tests and wrote some medications for me. Thank you very much.

Intervention

Did you report all current concerns you have been reporting to me, such as: 'swollen feet, shortness of breath, absence of menses for over six months, occasional absence of urine or strong amber brown urine and racing heart'?

Patient

Yes, I reported but the doctor said all those concerns will be addressed after the test.

Intervention

Did they take vital signs and see the swollen feet?

Patient

No, today they just saw me, but also the machine was broken so I could not be scheduled for a sonogram this week. But I have to find the medication they prescribed to me because the hospital pharmacy did not have the medication. [Weeks later] I am getting worse, it is getting difficult to walk, I am very weak, I cannot stand or walk on the hospital long lines so I have to find someone with transportation then I will go back for the tests […] We finally we have the tests done and I will share them with you.

Intervention

Almost a week from the last message I cannot reach her, I get a message from a family member who read my text to her saying 'she was hospitalized due to severe pain, she has been put on a strong pain medication and now she has been discharged but she sleeps throughout, she cannot walk or eat and needs to go to the hospital for pain medication because she wakes up crying in severe pain'.

Final stage
Desperately I am struggling to locate palliative care in the city from this end [....] no stone left unturned, sibling calling me crying and hoping there is something I could do [...] we are all losing hope [...] Christmas came [...] New Year came [...] she was no longer with us.

And so the battle that no one prepares for ended; revealing the dysfunctional and weak healthcare structure and system in another resource-poor country. It is a social catastrophe. Cancer is still a death sentence in our land, how many more deaths should we witness my dear brothers and sisters; how long should we continue to share sad stories and pain as we admit to our failure in saving lives in our lands. We need to set our communities free, free from this cancer epidemic, lack of awareness, education, resources, services, expertise and infrastructure. Collaboration can make a difference in strengthening or reforming our healthcare system, and prevent needless suffering and deaths.

Harriet Shangarai

***

Cameroon is a beautiful country famous for producing world-class soccer players and infectious 'makossa' music. It has been described as 'all Africa in one country' or 'Africa in miniature', boasting some of the richest and most diverse wildlife—a dreamland for safari lovers, eco tourists, hikers and culture seekers. As in other developing countries, cancer is rising devastatingly here, with new patients estimated in the tens of thousands each year, in contrast to the dearth of infrastructure to deal with it. With a population of over 22 million, Cameroon only has cancer centers at Yaoundé General Hospital and Douala General Hospital. However, at present, only Douala has a functional radiotherapy facility. Constraints in patients' access to cancer treatment (radiotherapy, chemotherapy and surgical services) present a significant challenge. The regulatory body (the National Radiation Protection Agency (NRPA)) has been mandated through laws and regulations to regulate all ionizing radiation sources and the protection of people and environment against ionizing radiation hazards. There are only two radiation oncologists and three certified medical physicists in the whole country, with one of them working with the NRPA. It is hoped here that with the help of international medical physics associations, the International Atomic Energy Agency (IAEA), the World Health Organization (WHO) and non-profit organizations, together with the Cameroon ministries of Public Health/Scientific Research/Higher Education, the fight against cancer will be taken to a new and improved level through global collaboration.

Collaborations could help to:

1. increase the capacity for cancer diagnosis in the areas of pathology, radiology and nuclear medicine by ensuring the availability of qualified human resources (professionals and technicians) and appropriate equipment (echography, mammography, CT scan and MRI);

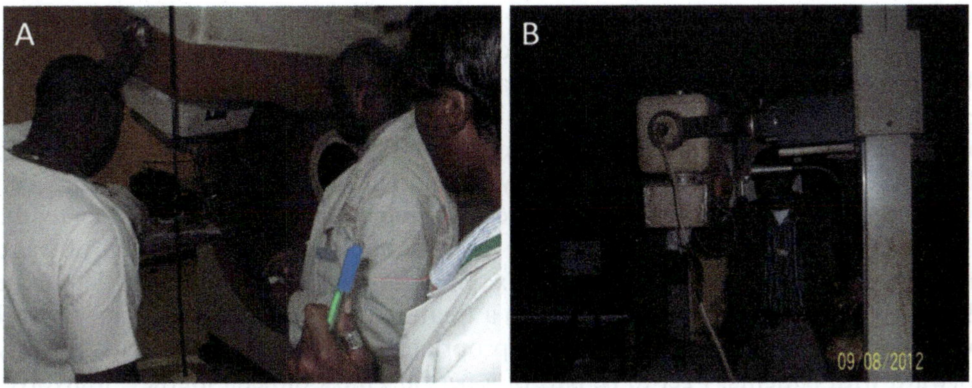

Figure 0.1. (A) Cobalt-60 radiotherapy machine being used without a treatment-planning system; (B) an x-ray machine installed in 1965 is still being used for diagnostic imaging.

2. establish a national radiotherapy plan covering the medium- and long-term and increase radiotherapy capacity in the short-term at the two existing centres (Yaoundé and Douala) by addressing all relevant areas (staffing, equipment, quality assurance programmes and maintenance policy);
3. perform regular quality control of equipment and ensure regular maintenance and servicing;
4. standardize treatment protocols for the most common cancers in Cameroon;
5. establish adequate radiation protection measures for personnel and patients, in particular in the brachytherapy unit of the Douala General Hospital, in compliance with national legislation and conditions imposed by the regulatory body, and take necessary actions to ensure that all radiology, radiotherapy and nuclear medicine departments in Cameroon have a valid licence issued by the NRPA;
6. foster education, research and training: education, research and training programs should accompany the general policy of cancer management and all relevant speciality programs in medical and non-medical fields should be initiated at the local universities to provide the required human resources;
7. foster palliative care: revise the current legislation on opioids to cover opioid supply, storage and prescription, and establish a list of essential medicines for palliative care (including oral preparations of morphine and other essential analgesics) in line with the WHO Essential Medicines in Palliative Care list.

The photographs in figure 0.1 highlight the disparities in cancer care services and why Cameroon could benefit from global radiation oncology.

Richard Ndi Samba

***

A typical day for me in the clinic

I am a young clinical oncologist (both radiation and medical oncology). The exciting thing about my job is the simple fact that I do not have a typical day at the clinic. Each day poses a new challenge, a learning opportunity and, more importantly, an opportunity to make a difference in another person's life. I care for patients with different emotional and physical needs. We would normally discuss the patients at a tumor board with colleagues from other disciplines before patients come to the clinic. At the new case clinic, I review patient histories and the results of basic investigations done, perform physical examinations, stage the patients, determine the best management and, finally, set up a treatment plan. In the follow-up clinic, I perform physical examinations, order appropriate investigations and discuss the way forward with patients. I get to be part of a person's most difficult journey, it involves sharing good news and sometimes bad news, tackling myths about cancer, radiotherapy and reassuring my patients. Listening and empathy are key to my job; the majority of our patients have to travel from distant regions to the only cancer institute currently providing radiotherapy.

The greatest challenges I face

1. Patients and society in general have low awareness about cancer and cancer prevention.
2. Limited availability of resources such as treatment machines, CT scans, laboratory equipment, etc.
3. No population-based cancer registry.
4. Balancing clinical work, teaching responsibilities and research.

What can be done to help me do my job better

I need more training on research, with opportunities to see and learn from other, more advanced, cancer institutes. We all have something to learn from each other. We all have something to offer. We speak the same language: science. Young scientists like me want to be part of the global science community. *Our ideas, knowledge and skills should not be limited by circumstances or by geographical location now that communication has been made so easy.*

International collaborations have opened doors for mentorship, exchange programs, telemedicine, visiting lecturers and research partnership. And these collaborations have proven to be very beneficial in many areas, including education. Global health is a growing academic field, where high-income country faculty and students can work in low- and middle-income countries and learn about new cultures, settings and diseases, possibly developing the expertise to address existing and emerging challenges in health care. Global health has brought beneficial medical knowledge to low- and middle-income countries: expertise in health policy and planning from high-income settings has improved clinic and hospital infrastructure and medical practice.

Patient care has also improved through direct communication via telemedicine, enabling consultations with colleagues who have more expertise in the field.

Exchange programs have opened the way for doctors from developing countries to gain expertise and skills, hence improving patient care when they return home, while doctors from developed countries acquire experience of tropical diseases, and everyone benefits from the cultural interchange and exposure to a different environment.

There are many research questions that are yet to be answered and collaboration between scientists provides an important channel to access knowledge and expertise and apply them to local problems. An example of such a collaboration is the Training Health Researchers into Vocational Excellence in East Africa (THRiVE) program, which aims to improve regional research capacity by linking academic institutions from Uganda, Rwanda, Tanzania and Kenya. The number of experienced researchers in Africa is still quite small and such collaborations enable young and inexperienced researchers from developing countries to obtain mentors from developed countries who can assist them in developing their research careers. Another advantage of collaborative research is that it can lead to the development of scientific facilities (such as laboratories), cancer registries, protocols, statistical expertise, databases and management expertise. It can also provide access to foreign sources of funding for researchers in developing countries and help young researchers to publish research and present their work at international conferences.

My inspiration for working in oncology, a medical area that many people believe is only about pain and death
I have always wanted to make a difference in people's lives and having a father who was one of the first pioneers in the fight against cancer in our country inspired me to join in the fight.

Mamsau Ngoma, Ocean Road Cancer Institute

***

When I was growing up, we had a breast cancer patient in our neighbourhood, who was frequently visited by a traditional healer. Sometimes she would lie outside for the Sun to dry out the wounds on her breast. For many poor people like her, with nowhere else to go, traditional healers are often the first and last line of defense against the most contagious and debilitating diseases. In her quest to seek better healthcare elsewhere, outside a country with few or no treatment options for her, she died on the way. As kids, her situation was incomprehensible to us, and there were many stories circulating about her illness.

Years later, with this experience at the back of my mind, Medical Physicists in the Diaspora for Africa (MephidA) was founded to fight against cancer in Africa. Intensifying global oncology collaborations in cancer care research and education would be a game changer, especially for sub-Saharan Africa, where the cancer-care disparities are huge. It would bring in diverse views, ideas and concepts that would certainly stimulate and catalyze our endeavors to help improve cancer care in sub-Sahara Africa, thereby promoting horizontal technical cooperation and the sustainability of existing cancer care centres. It would also attract more international volunteers/mentors in the oncology domain and establish closer links between radiation oncology professionals at home and in the diaspora. Involving more Africans in the diaspora could help facilitate global health collaborations and greater access to quality cancer care for patients in underserved areas.

'Medical physicist' is not a recognized profession in most African nations and African oncology centers are less involved in the global oncology research/education network. This can be changed gradually, with more attention being paid to global oncology collaborations in cancer research and the recognition of medical physicist as a profession in those African countries where it is not yet recognized.

With an intensive and well-coordinated global collaborative effort in oncology, the whole will be worth more than the sum of its parts, and patients will not have to lie out in the Sun to dry out the cancer on their breasts.

Ernest Okonkwo, MephidA, Germany

Foreword

For a very long time it has been common belief that cancer is not the most urgent problem in low and middle income countries (LMIC) because they supposedly have other, more pressing, problems with communicable diseases, malnutrition, and what not. But the reality is that great progress in those regions is translating into a gradual and steady, albeit uneven, increase in life expectancy. So much so, that Cancer is now being recognized as the silent epidemic and addressing it is one of the goals of the new century, and radiation oncology is one of the principal tools in this effort. It is also known that better radiation oncology provides effective, better and more successful treatment of cancer.

Having had the privilege of working in medical physics, in the most technological of healthcare environments, I have learned to appreciate the complexity and the high cost of linear accelerators, and the ever more sophisticated hardware, software, processes, and associated equipment necessary for well trained personnel to deliver high quality treatment in a safe manner. But it took more than half a century of major developments to get us to where we are now, in the 'developed countries'.

I have also learned that professionals in radiation oncology in developing countries—physicians, medical physicists, radiation technologists, nurses—and all those that support them, organizationally and technically, face way greater challenges than those that we ever faced in North America. So how are our medical physicist colleagues, for example in Africa, going to catch up with these advances and help bring their institutions to the current level of practice?

Some of us have tried to make a difference at various points in our careers by reaching out across the borders to share what we know. In the process we also learned quite a bit about the concrete challenges in some places. Along the way we have formed the most rewarding bonds with colleagues while at the same time realized the massive scope of the problem. We also recognized that we don't have the luxury to take another half century to implement solutions. These solutions have to be scalable and affordable, and close collaboration with other professionals is essential. We also need to share knowledge and experience, in both directions, as this is a key to addressing the global cancer epidemic.

It is with this in mind that in 2015 my friend and colleague Wil Ngwa, a medical physicist at Brigham and Women's Hospital and a co-director at the Harvard based Global Health Catalyst, along with a great group of colleagues, organized a summit of professionals from particularly diverse backgrounds, but with a shared goal of addressing the silent cancer epidemic. The aim was to consider all that we know, and to chart a cooperative path to advance that goal.

I am most pleased to see that soon after that this book was written, detailing the key issues for anyone interested in eliminating global radiotherapy disparities. It is a great place to get the whole picture of radiation oncology in the framework of global health for those that want to participate in global health but are not sure how.

It frames education and training efforts as a way to take advantage of the lessons learned so far on the need, the challenges and the opportunities currently available for radiation oncology in a clear and accessible way. It covers in detail the state of radiation oncology global health collaborations and points to resources available. One of these is the use of information and communication technologies (ICTs) to close the space-time gap between regions at a very affordable monetary cost. I am happy to see this work as a living textbook for all of us who are eager to address the global silent epidemic.

Yakov Pipman, DSc
Forest Hills, NY, USA
Co-founder and President Elect—Medical Physicists Without Borders
Chair of Professional Relations Committee—International Organization of Medical Physics
Chair of International Educational Activities—American Association of Physicists in Medicine

***

It is well over 30 years since I spent two semesters as a medical student in northern Nigeria and then another as a sub-intern in Sierra Leone. At that time the level of interest displayed in low-income nations was low and limited to small research groups and some missionary ventures. Man-made or natural catastrophes, such as the then recent wars in Biafra and Bangladesh, sparked occasional interest but this was usually short-lived. Emergency aid was briefly abundant, but sustainable contributions to health and welfare were not. Maternal and infant mortality was shockingly high, infectious diseases dominant, and cancer simply not a consideration. I was stunned to see curable cancers, such as Hodgkin and Burkitt Lymphomas, go neglected and unchecked for want of radiation or simple chemotherapy. Numerically speaking, however, cancer could not begin to match with the more urgent medical priorities of the day.

It is now 2016 and the world has changed. Infectious diseases are less of a challenge and the populations of these nations are living longer; long enough for cancer to emerge as a new threat to the health of working age men and women. This alone brings it into the sights of governments and domestic health care agencies. At the same time cancer therapies are more effective and some, particularly radiation, can be offered at remarkably low cost. Most importantly, the world is shrinking. Air travel is easy, cell phones are ubiquitous, and of course the internet binds us all instantaneously. Where there used to be nearly 200 nations there is increasingly one world connected 24/7. As time and distance shrinks so the barriers between nations blur, and the interests of one become the interests of all. This altered dynamic has suddenly made the growing cancer problem of the low and middle-income countries (LMIC) a problem for all of us in the global oncology community and, for the first time in human history, we are empowered to do something about it.

I look with incredible optimism at the many levels at which a mobilization is taking place. Supranational organizations, such as the Union for International Cancer Control (UICC) and the (World Health Organization (WHO), are folding cancer into their priority lists and dedicating funding and attention. The International Atomic

Energy Agency (IAEA) is focused on training and equipping small nations with safe radiation therapy capability. Governments themselves have put cancer on the agenda and found a place for it alongside the more perennial issues of hunger, communicable diseases, pests, and war. The major radiation oncology societies such as ASTRO and ESTRO have international relations committees and can serve in several broad ways. Firstly, they are huge repositories of educational material and educational talent, which they now propose to share through the web. In addition they can be the sponsors of exchange programs between the developed nations and the LMINs. They, together with governments, are also capable of placing pressure on the vendors to reconsider the pricing of both drugs and equipment. Some nations, such as India, are taking matters into their own hands and developing their own low-cost cobalt machines and linear accelerators (the Bhabhatron Project).

Below the international radiation oncology professional societies are the charitable foundations, small and large, who are now receptive to cancer projects. *Radiating Hope* and *Africans in the Diaspora* are two such examples, but the hope for the future is to engage the foundations of major benefactors many of whom are following the Bill Gates and Warren Buffet 'Giving Pledge'. The principal medical institutions of the developed nations have a new awareness of their global responsibilities, which, they now appreciate, work both ways. In developing fraternal relationships with hospitals in Africa or South America they not only increase the sum total of health of the world directly, but also give their young physicians extraordinary training and research opportunities. Many institutions, inspired by the writings and practices of Paul Farmer, see the return on investment in such relationships. A pairing of institutions is now taking place, not only through the traditional route of episodic exchange visits and material donation, but also through webcast conferences and tumor boards. This is a form of communication that is both inexpensive and invaluable. Many examples of 'twinned' institutions now exist, such as the Partners institutions in Boston with Botswana and the University of California at San Diego with Senegal, and it is to be hoped that these exemplary models will proliferate widely.

Finally, the most important ingredient will be the new generation of inspired young medical professionals. In the USA radiation oncology builds electives into its training and many are now seeking positions in LMIC funded either by their institutions, by the ASTRO Global Scholars Program, or by themselves. While they may not be able to do much on their own in their early visits, they return excited and empowered to become the new standard bearers of the global oncology movement. Indeed, at many academic institutions global health is seen as a legitimate academic pursuit with opportunities to blaze a real academic career path. The young physician and physicists' blogs and their social networks, propagate their enthusiasm, beat the drum, and prick the conscience of the specialty. Social media are uniquely powerful tools to raise awareness, drive action at the group and individual level, and to 'crowd-fund' projects. As I write, a 'Hack-a-Thon' is taking place in Boston to bring together innovators from technical colleges, health care providers, and field professionals, to brainstorm new affordable solutions for medical problems in the LMIC. The new media are stimulating creativity and bringing together unlikely partners in new combinations. The oncology journals, though 'old media' are still read with respect, and when they too start raising a global health message then it is clear that the message has become mainstream.

This eBook represents a first attempt to bind together in one place the projects and thoughts of the global radiation oncology community. It presents the insights of many engaged individuals, showing how far we have come, and how far we have yet to go. I have never been more optimistic about the prospects of making a radical difference in those nations that have no, or minimal, cancer care because the ingredients are all there. The societies and agencies are active and see this as a priority. The institutions and the new generation of volunteers are ready and can be scaled up considerably. The Internet is the 'secret sauce' that will make this contemporary endeavor succeed where previous attempts have been sporadic and half-hearted. Radiotherapy will be our tool, but the energy and creativity of the youthful radiation oncology community will be our fuel.

Anthony Zietman
Editor-in-Chief, *International Journal of Radiation Oncology*Biology*Physics*
Jenot W. and William U. Shipley Professor of Radiation Oncology,
Radiation Oncology, Harvard Medical School
Associate Director, Radiation Oncology Residency Program,
Massachusetts General Hospital

Acknowledgements

The authors would like to thank those who participated in the 2015 Global Health Catalyst Cancer Summit at Harvard Medical School and the International Medical Physics Symposium at the 2014 American Association of Physicists in Medicine conference. The useful discussions and model initiatives highlighted at these meetings are helping to generate/share new knowledge that is crucial for the emerging field of global radiation oncology.

Author biographies

Twalib Ngoma

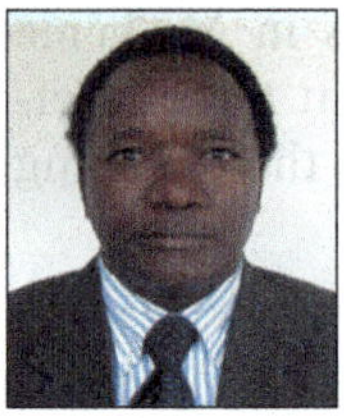

Professor Twalib Ngoma is a consultant clinical oncologist working at the Muhimbili University of Health and Allied Sciences (MUHAS), Tanzania. He founded the Ocean Road Cancer Institute (ORCI) in Tanzania and was the Executive Director of ORCI from 1996 to 2014. He has dedicated much of his career to improving oncology services in Tanzania and globally. He received the 2009 Nazli Gad-el-Mawla Award from the International Network for Cancer Treatment and Research (INCTR) for outstanding contributions to cancer control made by an individual from a country with limited resources and he was the 2015 Harvard Global Health Catalyst Award winner as the Africa Ambassador.

Wilfred Ngwa

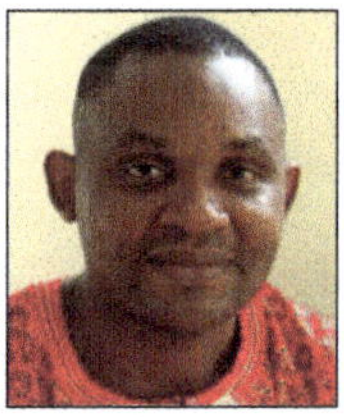

Wilfred Ngwa is the Director of the Global Health Catalyst program at Dana Farber/Harvard Cancer Center and a professor of radiation oncology and faculty medical physicist at Harvard Medical School and the University of Massachusetts. He also currently holds an international guest professorship at the University of Heidelberg, Germany. He has published two books and won a number of awards and prizes, including the 2015 BRIght Futures Prize for innovative new technology designed for use during radiotherapy to kill cancer cells that have spread to other parts of the body.

IOP Publishing

Chapter 1

Introduction to radiation oncology global health

The chance for a cure, the chance to live, should no longer remain an accident of geography.

Felicia Knaul *et al* [1]

1.1 Global radiation oncology defined

Cancer is a leading cause of death worldwide [2], a growing global pandemic characterized by the development of abnormal cells in the body that divide uncontrollably with the ability to spread through, infiltrate and destroy normal body tissue. Over 90% of cancer deaths are caused by the spread of cancer cells to other parts of a patient's body, which makes the disease more difficult to treat effectively.

In radiation oncology, ionizing radiation, usually in the form of x-rays, gamma rays, protons, or electrons, is employed to treat cancer. The ultimate goal of radiation therapy (RT) is to maximize the dose/damage to the cancer cells while minimizing any damage to healthy tissue. In developed countries, RT is used in the treatment of over 50% of cancer patients, to cure localized disease, palliate symptoms, and control disease in incurable cancers [2]. In developing countries, millions do not have access to RT services. With RT being a major part of cancer treatment, a growing number of radiation oncology health professionals, students and even retirees are rising up against the growing global scourge of cancer and participating in radiation oncology global health.

The Executive Board of the Consortium of Universities for Global Health (CUGH) developed the following definition for global health, as published in *The Lancet* in 2009 [3]:

> Global health is an area for study, research, and practice that places a priority on improving health and achieving equity in health for all people worldwide.

doi:10.1088/978-0-7503-1224-0ch1

> Global health emphasizes transnational health issues, determinants, and solutions; involves many disciplines within and beyond the health sciences and promotes interdisciplinary collaboration; and is a synthesis of population-based prevention with individual-level clinical care.

This definition distinguished global health from *international health*, which focuses on health issues in countries other than one's own, especially low- and middle-income countries (LMIC). It also distinguished global health from *public health,* which focuses on issues that affect the health of the population of a particular community or country, and where the development and implementation of solutions does not usually require global cooperation. All the same, the CUGH definition does recognize that global health has areas of overlap with the more established disciplines of public health and international health, and that all three share the following characteristics: 'priority on a population-based and preventive focus; concentration on poorer or vulnerable underserved populations; multidisciplinary and interdisciplinary approaches; emphasis on health as a public good, the importance of systems and structures; and the participation of several stakeholders' [3].

Also writing in *The Lancet* in 2010 [4], Friedman *et al,* a working group of the Association of Schools of Public Health Global Health Committee, noted that global health is often perceived as international aid, with technologies and interventions flowing from the wealthier developed countries of the Global North to the poorer countries of the Global South. Friedman *et al* offered a more nuanced and contemporary perspective, emphasizing interdependence and recognizing the many contributions from both resource-rich and resource-poor nations.

In 2014, in a seminal global health editorial in the *International Journal of Radiation Oncology • Biology • Physics*, Anthony Zietman espoused the need for greater participation of radiation oncology health professionals in global health, while highlighting the work of a number of global radiation oncology leaders and institutions [5]–[10]. Here, radiation oncology health professionals include: radiation oncologists (physicians), radiation oncology nurses, medical physicists, dosimetrists, radiation therapists and associated social workers at all levels. The participation of these health professionals in international collaborations in radiation oncology care, research and education, 'with priority on improving health and achieving equity in health for all people worldwide', essentially defines the emerging field of global radiation oncology.

1.2 The need for global radiation oncology

Meeting at the US National Institutes of Health (NIH), American Nobel Prize-winning scientist, Harold Varmus, and other country leaders concluded that successful campaigns to control cancer and improve current strategies will increasingly depend on concerted international collaborations [11]. Highlighting the urgent need for such collaborations, the World Health Organization (WHO) 2014 *Cancer Report* [12] described the growing global burden of cancer as alarming, a major obstacle to human development and well-being, with an increasing annual economic cost of over

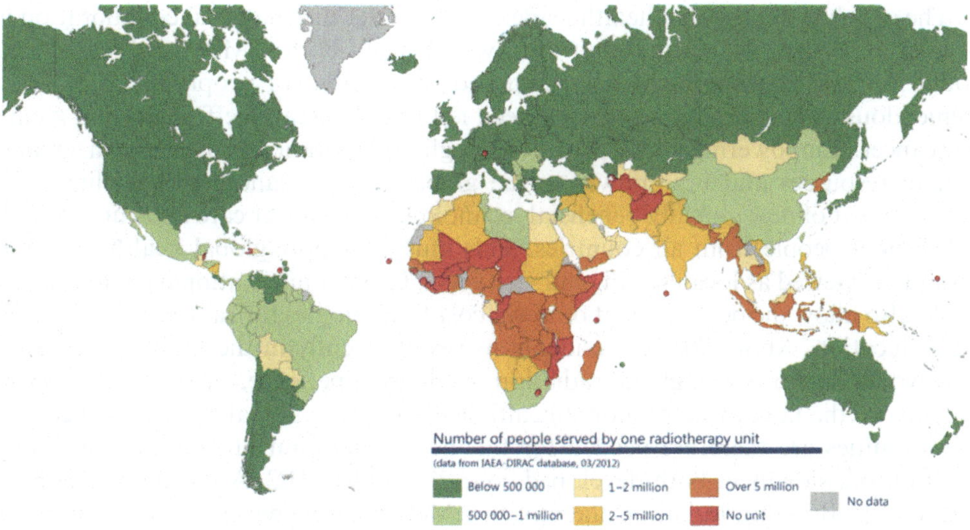

Figure 1.1. Global disparities in RT services. Reproduced with permission from the IAEA.

1.16 trillion US dollars. The report also highlighted major global cancer disparities, with over 60% of the 14 million new cases and 70% of 8.2 million deaths per year occurring in LMIC, some of which, sadly, are the least capable of dealing with cancer without some form of collaboration. The major disparities in cancer deaths are, in part, a reflection of the poignant underlying disparities in radiation oncology services (figure 1.1).

As figure 1.1 shows, the situation is particularly bad in LMIC in Africa, Asia and Latin America. For example, radiotherapy, which is needed in the treatment of over 50% of cancer patients [13], is not available in about half of Africa's 54 countries [14]. In Asian countries like India, many centers across the country do not have access to radiotherapy, with an average 2–5 million people per radiotherapy machine (compared with fewer than 250 000 people per machine in high-income countries) [15].

In LMIC, the range of radiotherapy needs which are currently covered varies from between 0% and 3–4% in low-income countries up to 59–79% in upper-middle-income countries in Europe and Central Asia [16]. According to Zubizaretta *et al* [16], the estimated number of additional radiation oncologists, medical physicists, dosimetrists and radiation therapists needed is over 43 000.

While the situation is worse in LMIC in Africa and Asia, the provision of radiotherapy facilities, equipment and trained staff is also inadequate in LMIC in South America. Furthermore, the first comprehensive analysis of DIrectory of RAdiotherapy Centres (DIRAC) data for Europe showed a substantial disparity in the availability and organization of radiotherapy services between countries, with a need to expand and modernize radiotherapy equipment in eastern and southeastern European countries [17].

The conclusion of global health leaders that greater international collaboration is needed [11] also recognized that this will benefit both LMIC and developed countries. For example, until now, hundreds of millions of people in LMIC with tremendous potential have essentially been left out of research efforts to find a cure for cancer. Empowering these people through collaborations can unleash greater human resources and brainpower in the global war on cancer and facilitate the development of new globally beneficial technologies for cancer care and cures, which will benefit people from all countries. This illustrates how global health can, and should, be viewed as local health, and vice versa. Greater international collaboration could also allow the development of lower cost technologies for cancer care, research and education. About 90% of residents surveyed recently in the USA [6] said that they would like to have a global radiation oncology experience, which could prepare them to be the next cadre of global health leaders. More global radiation oncology opportunities are therefore needed for this next generation of radiation oncology health professionals in both developed countries and LMIC. As Anthony Zietman put it [10], 'Bringing radiation therapy to LMIC is an increasingly global need or responsibility'. It would benefit global security and economic development. A recent *Lancet* study [2] demonstrated the substantial health and economic benefits that can be derived from investing in radiotherapy, especially in LMIC.

1.3 Growing interest and activity in global radiation oncology

A seminal article by Zietman *et al* [5]–[10] in the *International Journal of Radiation Oncology • Biology • Physics* inspired greater discussion of global health and health strategies at different levels, which could help address the growing global cancer burden and the tragic disparities in radiation oncology. The increase in publications and activity in recent years reflects the recent upsurge of interest in global radiation oncology, highlighting the need for greater action at all levels, from volunteers, individual hospitals, professional societies such as the American Society for Radiation Oncology (ASTRO), the European Society for Radiotherapy and Oncology (ESTRO) and the American Association for Physicists in Medicine (AAPM), supranational bodies and governments [10].

1.3.1 Volunteer level

Numerous volunteers from radiation oncology departments are rising up and reaching beyond their borders to participate in global radiation oncology, with many self-funding their participation and even using their vacation time for this. There are also currently opportunities for final year residents and faculty to participate in the Health Volunteers Overseas program associated with the American Society of Clinical Oncology. The upsurge of interest from radiation oncology residents [6] has also led many to begin choosing global radiation oncology career paths. Cognizant of the growing need for global radiation oncology and the upsurge of interest in this area, the ASTRO/ARRO Global Health Scholars (GHS) program is now helping to support senior residents interested in global health to work on a resident-designed clinical, outreach/educational or research project in LMIC. The GHS program provides scholarships that allow residents to become immersed in the different modalities of cancer care available in LMIC. It also helps them to develop a greater appreciation for the culture and attitudes related to cancer care, research and education. Such experience fosters a global perspective on oncology and encourages further outreach. As Thompson *et al* [18] note, such global health exchanges must grow beyond 'medical tourism' and should instead continue to nurture the roots of a more robust international care network, with opportunities for cancer care, research and education. Such exchange programs produce benefits for everyone involved, with a bidirectional commitment to knowledge sharing, evidence development and resource exchange.

1.3.2 Professional society level

At the professional society level, ASTRO and its associated journal, the *Red Journal* already recognizes that its mission cannot be limited to the USA [8], and must extend across international borders to help lead global improvements in the quality and safety of radiation oncology care. ASTRO can have a broad impact by drawing on the expertise, time and volunteerism of the many ASTRO members who are interested in and committed to international outreach and education. ASTRO's wealth of electronic and archived educational materials provide complementary resources for these efforts by enabling virtual long-distance and more cost-effective pathways for international education. The *Red Journal* has also increased efforts to advance global health [10].

Meanwhile, ESTRO is also boosting its global radiation oncology efforts through its Health Economics in Radiation Oncology (HERO) project, which helps European national radiotherapy societies to strengthen the profession in their respective countries. ESTRO [19] also signaled early support for the Global Task Force on Radiotherapy for Cancer Control (GTFRCC) [9], and ESTRO's associated journal, the *Green Journal* established a Global Radiation Oncology Collaboration in Education (GRaCE) program [20]. In establishing GRaCE, common areas of educational interest and need were defined, which included the development of new competency statements and assessment tools, and the application of these tools. Such a program provides a valuable mechanism to ensure that training programs are up to date, and to enhance radiation oncology education, through sharing resources and expertise.

Another professional society, the AAPM, inherently sponsors, or co-sponsors, a variety of educational and training programs in cooperation with medical physics organizations throughout the world [21]. The AAPM currently provides the following educational resources for medical physicists in developing countries: Proceedings of the AAPM Summer Schools, Continuing Education Programs from the Annual Meetings and selected AAPM Task Group Reports. More and more sessions are being organized on global health and radiation oncology. One is likely to see increased activity in the coming years.

Close relationships between these radiation oncology professional societies hold the promise that global radiation oncology efforts can at least be complemented by educational efforts. The Harvard Global Health Catalyst summit is working to facilitate such close relationships and knowledge sharing. There are also an increasing number of sessions at the professional society annual conferences that bring together global health leaders in radiation oncology from these different professional societies to work together, share knowledge, or initiate more concerted efforts. At the 2014 AAPM conference in Texas, Ngwa *et al* [22] began one such concerted effort to leverage information and communication technologies (ICTs) in catalyzing global health collaborations in radiation oncology and enhancing the effectiveness of other global radiation oncology programs. This led to or helped spawn a number of tangible global radiation oncology initiatives, including the emerging UPENN–Harvard–Tanzania education and training program powered by ICTs and led by Stephen Avery and Twalib Ngoma at Muhimbili University of Health and Allied Sciences (MUHAS) [23], [24]. Erno Sajo has also begun a University of Massachusetts Lowell (UML)–University of Heidelberg partnership that allows medical physics courses from Heidelberg to be recognized directly in UML, and hence the USA [25]. It is evident that these efforts will only grow in number, impact and scale. The Global Health Catalyst Summit plans to catalyze more such efforts, including the establishment of a virtual global radiation oncology education center of excellence in partnership with ASTRO, AAPM and the African Organization for Research and Training in Cancer (AORTIC).

1.3.3 Institutional or non-profit organization level

While professional societies are increasing global radiation oncology efforts, it is beyond the scope of a professional society to manage or maintain individual physician-to-physician and institution-to-institution relationships, which are critical to cultivating global radiation oncology that is tailored to the specific needs of the local treatment teams, institutions and environments. As Mayr *et al* noted, personalized relationships, which bolster long-term one-on-one exchanges, are just as important and can overcome economic, linguistic, or, in some regions, IT connectivity barriers [8]. Institutional level efforts are, therefore, also beginning to grow in quantity and quality, e.g. in twinning partnerships between developed country and LMIC institutions. Examples include the University of Sydney (Australia) and Myanmar partnership, where the Australian partner has helped bring about a major improvement in radiation oncology health services in Myanmar, significantly reducing the waiting time for people seeking treatment for cancer [26]. The BOTSwana Oncology Global Outreach program (BOTSOGO) [27] between Botswana and MGH/Harvard is another example, which will be further discussed along with others in subsequent chapters.

Meanwhile, a number of non-profit organizations with global radiation oncology mission statements are also emerging. One example is Medical Physicists without Borders [23], whose mission is to support activities that will yield effective and safe use of physics and technologies in medicine through advising, training, demonstrating and/or participating in medical physics-related activities, especially in LMIC. In Europe, the Mephida (Medical Physicists in Diaspora (Europe) for Cancer Care in Africa) Medical Foundation is another emerging independent non-profit organization with a novel approach to advancing and improving cancer care in Africa through medical physics [28]. A further example of a non-profit organization is Radiating Hope, where Fisher *et al* have been leading global radiation oncology work in a number of African countries [29]. Some of their commendable work in Senegal has been performed in partnership with Arno J Mundt [10, 29], at the University of California, San Diego. Another emerging salient non-profit organization is the International Cancer Expert Corps (ICEC), with a mission to reduce mortality and improve the quality of life for people with cancer in LMIC and other regions worldwide. The ICEC addresses this mission through a mentoring network of cancer professionals who work with local and regional in-country groups to develop and sustain expertise for better cancer care [30].

1.3.4 Government level

As Anthony Zietman noted [10], governments have a major role to play in terms of financial aid as well as symbolic political support. The President's Emergency Plan for AIDS Relief (PEPFAR), an initiative launched by the US government, is an example of a program that has made a tremendous impact in curbing diseases such as HIV/AIDS. Collaborations that involve governments, such as that between Partners in Health and the government of Rwanda [31], also help to ensure sustainability. Many LMIC governments are developing cancer control programs with the support of the IAEA Program of Action in Cancer Therapy (PACT) program and other organizations. Such government-level involvement is an important component in advancing global oncology efforts. It also helps to ensure synergistic efforts with optimal use of resources.

1.3.5 Supranational level

At the supranational level, the IAEA PACT program has been a major global radiation oncology leader, making substantial high-impact investments to improve the cancer situation in LMIC [2], [32]–[34]. Established in 2004, the program's goal is to fully realize the public health impact obtained through global partnerships in cancer control and technology transfer in radiation medicine. PACT strives to build global partnerships to confront the cancer crisis in developing countries, working with WHO and others.

In addition, under the outstanding leadership of Mary Gospodarowicz, the Union for International Cancer Control (UICC) established a Global Task Force on Radiotherapy for Cancer Control (GTFRCC) [9] to unite the cancer community to reduce the global cancer burden, promote greater equity and integrate cancer control into the world health and development agenda. The task force was challenged to provide the world with a clear assessment of the cancer treatment radiotherapy shortfall, raise awareness, facilitate planning, attract investment and improve global access to this powerful, effective and critical component of cancer treatment. The work led to the publication of the *Lancet* Commission report in 2015 [2]. The report highlights the need to respond urgently and speak with one voice to advocate immediate investment in radiation oncology facilities and the training of radiation therapy professionals to close the cancer divide [9]. A Young Leaders Program of the GTFRCC has also been initiated (GlobalRT) to work to make radiotherapy a global health priority [35].

Other exemplary global oncology efforts include work on radiation therapy quality assurance in clinical trials [36]–[38] and the Health Economics in Radiation Oncology project [39]. Another example is the Cross-Border Collaboration in Oncology Model for United States–Mexico Border Health [40, 41]. These examples of a significant increase of activity and interest in global radiation oncology are by no means exhaustive, but they highlight this burgeoning area as more and more people in radiation oncology reach beyond their borders [42] to make a much-needed impact on global health. These are exciting times for a growing field that can make a major impact in addressing the global burden of cancer, preventing needless suffering and deaths and eliminating global cancer disparities.

References

[1] Knaul F M, Frenk J and Shulman L 2011 Access to cancer care and control in developing countries. Closing the cancer divide: a blueprint to expand access in low and middle income countries, Harvard Global Equity Initiative, Boston, MA

[2] Atun R *et al* 2015 Expanding global access to radiotherapy *Lancet Oncol.* **16** 1153–86

[3] Koplan J P, Bond T C, Merson M H, Reddy K S, Rodriguez M H, Sewankambo N K and Wasserheit J N (Consortium of Universities for Global Health Executive) 2009 Towards a common definition of global health *Lancet* **373** 1993–5

[4] Fried L P, Bentley M E, Buekens P, Burke D S, Frenk J J, Klag M J and Spencer H C 2010 Global health is public health *Lancet* **375** 535–7

[5] Zietman A 2014 Bringing radiation therapy to underserved nations: an increasingly global responsibility in an ever-shrinking world *Int. J. Radiat. Oncol. Biol. Phys.* **89** 440–2

[6] Dad L, Shah M M, Mutter R, Olsen J, Dominello M, Miller S M, Fisher B, Lee N and Komaki R 2014 Why target the globe?: Four-year report (2009–2013) of the Association of Residents in Radiation Oncology Global Health Initiative *Int. J. Radiat. Oncol. Biol. Phys.* **89** 485–91

[7] Coleman C N *et al* 2014 Bringing cancer care to the underserved globally: a challenging problem for which radiation oncology can pioneer novel solutions *Int. J. Radiat. Oncol. Biol. Phys.* **89** 443–5

[8] Mayr N A *et al* 2014 International outreach: what is the responsibility of ASTRO and the major international radiation oncology societies? *Int. J. Radiat. Oncol. Biol. Phys.* **89** 481–4

[9] Jaffray D A and Gospodarowicz M 2014 Bringing global access to radiation therapy: time for a change in approach *Int. J. Radiat. Oncol. Biol. Phys.* **89** 446–7

[10] Zietman A 2014 Bringing radiation therapy to underserved nations: an increasingly global responsibility in an ever-shrinking world *Int. J. Radiat. Oncol. Biol. Phys.* **89** 440–2

[11] Varmus H and Kumar H S 2013 Addressing the growing international challenge of cancer: a multinational perspective *Sci. Transl. Med.* **5** 175 cm2

[12] Stewart B W and Wild C P 2014 *World Cancer Report* 2014 (IARC)

[13] Samiei M 2013 Challenges of making radiotherapy accessible in developing countries *Cancer Control* 85–94

[14] Abdel-Wahab M, Bourque J M, Pynda Y, Izewska J, Van der Merwe D, Zubizarreta E and Rosenblatt E 2013 Status of radiotherapy resources in Africa: an International Atomic Energy Agency analysis *Lancet Oncol.* **14** e168–175

[15] Pramesh C S *et al* 2014 Delivery of affordable and equitable cancer care in India *Lancet Oncol.* **15** e223–233

[16] Zubizarreta E H, Fidarova E, Healy B and Rosenblatt E 2015 Need for radiotherapy in low and middle income countries—the silent crisis continues *Clin. Oncol. (R. Coll. Radiol.)* **27** 107–14

[17] Rosenblatt E, Izewska J, Anacak Y, Pynda Y, Scalliet P, Boniol M and Autier P 2013 Radiotherapy capacity in European countries: an analysis of the DIrectory of RAdiotherapy Centres (DIRAC) database *Lancet Oncol.* **14** e79–86

[18] Thompson R F and Grover S 2015 A resident's perspective on global health rotations in radiation oncology *Int. J. Radiat. Oncol. Biol. Phys.* **93** 1165–6

[19] Poortmans P, Valentini V and Lievens Y 2015 Expanding global access to radiotherapy: the European Society for Radiotherapy and Oncology perspective *Lancet Oncol.* **16** 1148–9

[20] Turner S, Eriksen J G, Trotter T, Verfaillie C, Benstead K, Giuliani M, Poortmans P, Holt T, Brennan S and Potter R 2015 Establishing a global radiation oncology collaboration in education (GRaCE): objectives and priorities *Radiother. Oncol.* **117** 188–92

[21] AAPM 2016 *AAPM International Portal* www.aapm.org/international/default.asp

[22] Ngwa W *et al* 2015 Potential for information and communication technologies to catalyze global collaborations in radiation oncology *Int. J. Radiat. Oncol. Biol. Phys.* **91** 444–7

[23] Ngwa W *et al* 2016 Closing the Cancer Divide through Ubuntu: Information and Communication Technology Powered Models for Global Radiation Oncology *at press*

[24] Avery S, Kenton O, Bin Dachi J, Metz J and Ngwa W 2015 Radiation oncology solutions in Tanzania *Int. J. Radiat. Oncol. Biol. Phys.* **93** 961–9C2

[25] Medical physics education across continents: the UMass Lowell and Heidelberg University Joint Coordination Effort www.aapm.org/education/VL/vl.asp?id=3859

[26] Supporting radiation therapy clinical training in Myanmar http://sydney.edu.au/global-health/news-events/2015/news-story-48.php

[27] Efstathiou J A *et al* 2014 Addressing the growing cancer burden in the wake of the AIDS epidemic in Botswana: the BOTSOGO collaborative partnership *Int. J. Radiat. Oncol. Biol. Phys.* **89** 468–75 2014

[28] *Mephida* www.okonmedphys.com

[29] Fisher B J, Daugherty L C, Einck J P, Suneja G, Shah M M, Dad L K, Mutter R W, Wilkinson J B and Mundt A J 2014 Radiation oncology in Africa: improving access to cancer care on the African continent *Int. J. Radiat. Oncol. Biol. Phys.* **89** 458–61

[30] Coleman C N 2014 The international cancer expert corps: a unique approach for sustainable cancer care in low and lower-middle income countries *Front. Oncol.* **4** 333

[31] Binagwaho A, Wagner C M and Farmer P E 2016 A vision for global cancer medicine: pursuing the equity of chance *J. Clin. Oncol.* **34** 3–5

[32] Rosenblatt E, Zubizarreta E, Wondergem J, Fidarova E and Izewska J 2012 The International Atomic Energy Agency (IAEA): an active role in the global fight against cancer *Radiother. Oncol.* **104** 269–71

[33] Rosenblatt E, Acuna O and Abdel-Wahab M 2015 The challenge of global radiation therapy: an IAEA perspective *Int. J. Radiat. Oncol. Biol. Phys.* **91** 687–9

[34] Enwerem-Bromson N and Abdel-Wahab M 2015 Expanding global access to radiotherapy: the IAEA perspective *Lancet Oncol.* **16** 1151–2

[35] Rodin D, Yap M L and Hanna T P 2014 GlobalRT: building a new radiotherapy community *Lancet Oncol.* **15** 926

[36] Melidis C *et al* 2015 Global harmonization of quality assurance naming conventions in radiation therapy clinical trials *Int. J. Radiat. Oncol. Biol. Phys.* **91** 1115 (erratum)
[37] Melidis C *et al* 2014 Radiation therapy quality assurance in clinical trials—global harmonisation group *Radiother. Oncol.* **111** 327–9
[38] Melidis C *et al* 2014 Global harmonization of quality assurance naming conventions in radiation therapy clinical trials *Int. J. Radiat. Oncol. Biol. Phys.* **90** 1242–9
[39] Lievens Y and Grau C 2012 Health economics in radiation oncology: introducing the ESTRO HERO project *Radiother. Oncol.* **103** 109–12
[40] Jabbari S *et al* 2015 Cross-border collaboration in oncology: a model for United States–Mexico border health *Int. J. Radiat. Oncol. Biol. Phys.* **93** 472 (erratum)
[41] Jabbari S *et al* 2015 Cross-border collaboration in oncology: a model for United States–Mexico border health *Int. J. Radiat. Oncol. Biol. Phys.* **92** 509–11
[42] Elmore S N *et al* 2016 Global radiation oncology from the trainee perspective: a view from beyond the bunker *Int. J. Radiat. Oncol. Biol. Phys.* **94** 438–9

Chapter 2

Challenges and new opportunities in global radiation oncology

It always seems impossible until it's done.
Nelson Mandela [1]

2.1 Introduction

Despite the upsurge of interest in and growing activity for global health, there are a number of challenges that need to be addressed to facilitate greater participation and bolster the growing field of global radiation oncology. Some examples of these challenges are highlighted below.

2.2 Perceptions or lack of awareness

The alarming cancer statistics stand in stark contrast to an equally alarming lack of awareness, both locally and globally. A distressing illustration of this can be seen in many LMIC, where so many languages do not even have a word for cancer. If people are not aware of the disease, or do not have the right perception or appreciation of the problem, it goes without saying that they cannot develop an appropriate response. For example, most of Africa's over 2000 languages do not have a word for cancer [3]. So in these LMIC, many people die painfully of cancer and, sadly, have no idea what they died of, while others attribute the cause of death to something else. In areas more familiar with cancer, there is an adverse perception or a strong social stigma associated with the disease [4]; even young doctors do not want to specialize in oncology, a medical area that talks only about pain and death. The lack of cancer awareness and the stigmatization also mean that the overwhelming majority of patients only present late with the disease, when it is too late to cure them; the ensuing deaths then further reinforce the notion that cancer is

doi:10.1088/978-0-7503-1224-0ch2

essentially a death sentence. In some countries, there is also a long-standing perception that cancer is a systemic illness and that investment in local treatment modalities will not reduce death rates.

Regarding radiotherapy, people in some LMIC may be more afraid of radiation than they are of cancer. For example, in India many people call radiation therapy 'electrical current treatment', implying that it shocks, burns and can even kill [5], while in Tanzania people call radiotherapy 'fire treatment', and health workers tell patients that they are going to receive 'burn treatment'. On hearing this, patients become scared and question why on earth they should be punished by getting cancer in the first place and then be burnt before they die. As a result of this, some patients decide to abandon treatment altogether. Furthermore, there is often a perception that radiotherapy is too expensive an investment, or that other priorities in cancer care are more important, or that in the longer term newer treatments will replace radiotherapy and therefore the investment is not required. These adverse perceptions have limited investment in appropriate radiotherapy resources in many countries. While radiotherapy is perceived to be an expensive treatment modality, the facts speak otherwise. One radiation machine can treat thousands of cancer patients over many years. In fact, the recent *Lancet* Commission report [6] provided compelling evidence that investment in radiotherapy not only enables large numbers of cancer cases to be treated to save lives, but is also more cost-effective in the longer term and brings positive economic benefits.

There is opportunity here to promote greater cancer awareness education and evidenced-based advocacy. In many LMIC, it is not uncommon for women with breast cancer to be considered to be diminished in their femininity. Concerned about the possibility of being abandoned by their spouses when diagnosed with cancer, many decide not to look for care, or, if they do, to reject proper treatment. 'A woman is more than her breasts' is attributed to global health leader, Julio Frenk, who has championed major advances in cancer in Mexico with his wife Felicia Knaul. Messages and lessons such as these could be extended to benefit other LMIC.

Fortunately, some governments in LMIC are becoming more aware of the cancer threat. Efforts to support cancer research in developing nations, though still meager, are increasing. More cancer awareness and education in partnership with LMIC governments could help to change perceptions and bolster the political will required for greater investment in radiotherapy, beginning with infrastructure.

2.3 Infrastructure

In order to address the growing global cancer burden and effect the required productive and sustainable international collaborations, fundamental infrastructure is crucial. In a recent editorial [7], Petereit and Coleman highlighted the pivotal need to develop and sustain the infrastructure required for radiotherapy in LMIC. The IAEA recommends a teletherapy unit, a radiation oncologist, a medical physicist and two radiotherapists per 250 000 people [8]–[11]. Datta *et al* reported in 2014 that only four of the 139 LMIC have the requisite number of teletherapy units, and 55 (39.5%) have no radiation therapy facilities [12, 13].

In addition to requiring clinical infrastructure, the ability of LMIC scientists to carry out rigorous cancer research during collaborations depends on the availability of research infrastructure at both the institutional and national levels. As Adewole *et al* report [14], the availability of research infrastructure remains inadequate in most LMIC. Besides the challenges posed by limited laboratory infrastructure, the lack of research administration infrastructure is also a challenge. Research administration provides the necessary oversight and coordination of activity within an institution and sets the tone for fiscal responsibility, ensuring the appropriate use of research funds. However, there is still a severe lack of such administrative infrastructure in LMIC. Many researchers and engineers in LMIC also suffer from the long times they have to wait before research consumables or machine spare parts are delivered after purchase, given that many companies who supply these items are located in Europe and North America.

The lack or shortage of infrastructure in LMIC is an opportunity for new technologies to be developed that can make significant improvements to this challenging situation, which could also help populations in resource-rich countries. It is also an opportunity to establish greater partnerships with industry and an incentive to invest more in these LMIC. The US NIH announced a new funding opportunity: Cancer Detection, Diagnosis, and Treatment Technologies for Global Health. This initiative supports the development of cancer-relevant technologies suitable for use in LMIC. 'Specifically, the funding opportunity solicits applications for projects to adapt, apply, and validate existing or emerging technologies into a new generation of user-friendly, low-cost devices or assays that are clinically comparable to currently used technologies for imaging, *in vitro* detection/diagnosis, prevention or treatment of cancers in humans living in LMIC' [15]. This opportunity should also help spur physicists and other scientists across different disciplines to collaborate in developing lower-cost technologies for radiotherapy. More such funding opportunities are needed. Some of the emerging lower-cost technologies for radiotherapy are highlighted in chapter 5.

Greater investment in radiotherapy infrastructure and services will have tremendous economic benefits, not only enabling large numbers of cancer cases to be treated to save lives, but also bringing positive economic effects. The recent *Lancet* Commission report [6] estimates a net economic benefit of hundreds of billions of US dollars by 2035. For example, using the nominal cost model, with an expenditure of 265·2 million US dollars it could produce a net benefit of 278.1 billion US dollars in low-income countries, 38·5 billion US dollars in lower-middle-income countries and 239·3 billion US dollars in upper-middle-income countries.

2.4 Human resources and capacity

Another major challenge for successful and sustainable cancer management and global radiation oncology is the shortage in human capacity. In 2015, the number of additional radiation oncologists, medical physicists and radiation therapists needed was estimated to be 43 200 [8]. The dearth of infrastructure described above provides little incentive to train or develop human capacity, since the new people will not have the infrastructure they need to do their jobs. The shortage in human capacity is exacerbated by a number of other factors. These include a culture of silence and the strong social stigma associated with cancer [4]; there is little motivation for young doctors to specialize in oncology. The shortage in human capacity is also exacerbated by a brain drain. For example, in African LMIC, over 20 000 educated Africans leave the continent each year for greener pastures abroad [2]. Cognizant of the brain drain issue, the Harvard Global Health Catalyst (GHC) program has taken the opportunity to actively engage the resource-laden diaspora, turning the brain drain into a gain against cancer. This will provide further opportunities for more education/training activity to get more people involved in this field.

In general, the emerging field of global radiation oncology provides opportunities for the education/training of future radiation oncology health professionals who are focused on global health as part of the overall strategy for improving sustainable cancer care, research and education. Addressing the human resource shortages in LMIC could yield great dividends in the global war on cancer. It could bring thousands, if not tens of thousands, of people into cancer research, education and care. This would unleash unprecedented brainpower and human resources to address the growing cancer burden, advancing globally beneficial research and innovation that will save lives and drive economic development and global security.

Some have suggested that a targeted education and training plan should be developed with new career paths for work in LMIC and also in underserved areas within developed countries like the United States [16]. This effort could incorporate principles of cancer care and public health and address the scope of the challenges. For trainees, short-term initiatives might include seminars and workshops on global health, possibly in collaboration with schools of public health. After training, trainees could continue with some international experience in an LMIC, e.g. via short-term visits. The visiting trainee could spend time with all members of staff, including physicians, technicians, physicists, diagnostic imagers and administrators, to develop a better sense of the healthcare context. Education and training could then continue with the help of ICTs back at the home institution to maintain collaboration with the LMIC. The ICEC has also proffered the idea of senior residents in developed countries 'adopting a junior resident' in an LMIC and building a long-term relationship through tutoring, e-mail, video-conferencing and visits over the course of training. This ability to collaborate with LMIC healthcare staff and residents continuously could then lead to long-term professional collaborations, which could help sustain the global radiation oncology effort.

Overall, the human resource challenge could be complementarily addressed alongside the infrastructure problem discussed earlier in a comprehensive approach to global radiation oncology. Such capacity building would also engender radiation oncology health professionals in LMIC who can then further collaborate with developed country partners in more cancer education, research and care.

2.5 Finance/funding

One of the greatest challenges highlighted by global health leaders at the GHC summit was the limited funding available to support global oncology. In LMIC, relatively little funding is allocated for research. Meanwhile, in developed countries, the funding allocated to non-communicable diseases like cancer has traditionally been small compared to the funding for communicable diseases like HIV/AIDS (figure 2.1) [17]. This limited funding puts significant financial pressure on support for research and personnel in both LMIC and developed countries for global health work, including global radiation oncology.

The situation does provide opportunities for resource-rich countries to learn from resource-poor countries, because the latter are forced to optimize their return on every health care dollar with innovative solutions. Limited funding for global radiation oncology also provides opportunities for innovative financing mechanisms. Already some people are coming up with innovative funding mechanisms and even public–private partnerships that could help support/seed collaborations with LMIC in cancer [2, 18]. There are also opportunities for greater advocacy in this area, to encourage partner governments to invest more. Partnerships with local governments have an excellent record of helping to sustain global health activity, as the example of Partners in Health and the Rwanda Ministry of Health illustrates [19].

One of the innovative approaches highlighted at the Harvard summit that could be advocated for further, and which has been shown to be successful, is the tobacco tax. The Task Force on Innovative International Financing for Health Systems [20] included a recommendation to explore the technical viability of tobacco taxes as a solidarity levy for innovative financing for LMIC health systems. As a result of the working group's analysis, some complementary approaches were proposed for implementing the Task Force recommendation: a country approach and a global approach. In the country approach, increased tobacco taxes would provide the added benefit of decreasing tobacco use, which is a major cause of cancer, and therefore lead to improved population health. A recent WHO estimate showed that an increase of 50% in cigarette excise taxes in 22 of the 49 low-income countries would generate a total of 1.42 billion US dollars. The report noted that in LMIC like Congo, Laos or Vietnam, the extra revenue could be equivalent to an increase in current government expenditure of more than 25% (World Health Report 2010 [21]).

At the Harvard summit, another innovative financing approach that was discussed was that of crowdfunding for research, with possible support from the diaspora [2]. Given the tens of billions of US dollars in remittances, and more tens of billions in savings, the African diaspora, for example, has enormous potential to support global oncology efforts that would benefit their original countries. The crowdfunding approach is growing in popularity in developed countries like the USA, as seen in the many crowdfunding organizations, such as Rockethub, Kickstarter and others. Crowdfunding would be particularly beneficial for resource-poor settings, where even relatively small contributions can lead to many years of fruitful research for cancer researchers who would otherwise have no funding. Such crowdfunding can also be used to generate preliminary data to be more competitive when applying for funding, including international such as that provided by the US NIH. These preliminary data would also engender new hypotheses for more globally beneficial research and create greater visibility for LMIC researchers working with their developed-country peers to publish these data. Cancer research in LMIC will also help in driving public policy,

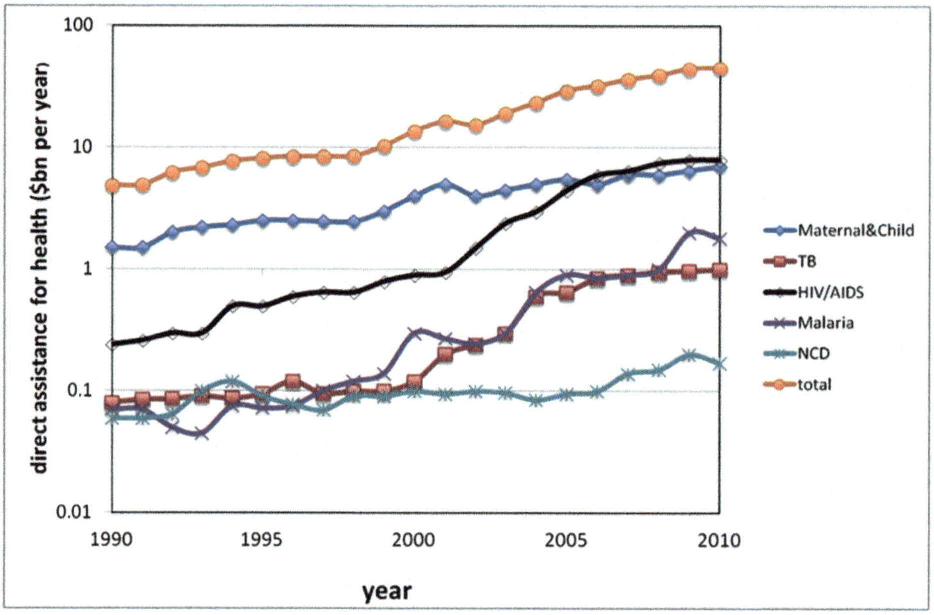

Figure 2.1. Trends in direct financial assistance for health measured in billions of US dollars per year with five of the principal areas of investment. TB: tuberculosis and NCD: non-communicable (non-infectious) diseases. Data taken from Murray *et al* [17].

changing perceptions, generating new knowledge and technologies for clinical translation and enabling participation in clinical trials, and it will benefit economic development. There are also opportunities for greater advocacy in this area, to have partner governments invest more in cancer care, research and education, which would help sustainability [17].

As mentioned previously, ARRO/ASTRO is now also providing opportunities via scholarships through its GHS program. Such support needs to be increased and other professional societies like the AAPM could also emulate this for medical physics trainees and faculty. There are also currently opportunities for final year residents and faculty to participate in ASCO's Health Volunteers Overseas program. This program recruits oncology physicians who can share their medical expertise and build sustainable relationships with physicians associated with cancer centers in LMIC. Participants can be involved in the teaching or training of staff and gain insights into the cancer center's management needs and challenges.

A private nongovernmental organization called Seed Global Health [22], founded by Vanessa Kerry, also helps provide financial opportunities to address the capacity/human resource challenge via the Global Health Service Partnership (GHSP) program. This innovative program sends US physicians and nurses to serve as faculty at medical and nursing schools in LMIC to increase the quantity and quality of graduates, thereby strengthening local health systems. The GHSP is a transformative collaboration between Seed Global Health and the Peace Corps, and is supported by the President's Emergency Plan for AIDS Relief [22]. Other organizations providing opportunities for training and global radiation oncology experience include the IAEA and Radiating Hope.

Another innovative financing approach, which was recently highlighted by the *Lancet* Oncology Commission report, includes guarantees by development banks [6]. Such guarantees by development banks can encourage private financing by minimizing risks in LMIC. It was reported that 4.5 billion US dollars in guarantees were provided by the World Bank Group in a year. These guarantees can be structured as partial risk guarantees to support private sector investment, including public–private partnerships. They can also support partial credit guarantees for commercial borrowing in support of public investment projects, amongst other things. The reduced risk of default provided by such guarantees improves a government's ability to borrow for investment. The guarantees can also allow governments to share the risks of investment in radiotherapy with the private sector.

2.6 Space–time challenge

A major challenge for converting the recent upsurge in global health interest [23] into more high-impact collaborations is the space–time factor. While many developed country health workers would like to collaborate with LMIC, the distances (space) they have to cover in travelling to LMIC can be a significant impediment. Given the busy schedules and little time people have, it is difficult to contribute to global health even when people want to, and this is especially the case in view of the lack of recognition global health still receives as part of professional/career development in radiation oncology.

For research collaborations across distances, it is also important that research tasks be clearly defined and owned by the individual scientists. When scientists are collocated they can informally observe and discuss tasks as they progress. This is more difficult to do across distances, and hence defining tasks and task responsibility clearly from the outset is vital. It can also be challenging to schedule meetings or tumor boards in geographically dispersed collaborations, since time zones, national holidays and organizational calendars may differ.

Advances in ICTs now offer opportunities to address the space–time challenge at a lower cost. ICTs have ushered in an unprecedented era where interactions with people across the globe are just a Skype login or cell phone call away. This includes interactions with partners in LMIC where cell phones are relatively ubiquitous, e.g. in Africa. These advances in ICTs can elide space and time, making it possible for radiation oncology health professionals in developed countries to participate in global health collaborations without necessarily travelling physically or having to take time off to do so. Ngwa *et al* recently highlighted the potential of ICTs to catalyze high-impact international collaborations in radiation oncology [23]. Such use of ICTs for global radiation oncology will be covered more expansively in chapter 5.

2.7 Bandwidth for use of ICTs

While ICTs have tremendous potential to help mitigate the space–time challenge and complement other face-to-face initiatives, this requires connectivity. Although broadband is increasingly available and the digital divide is a term that is no longer *en vogue*, more needs to be done to overcome the problem of bandwidth. Greater investment in broadband infrastructure will not only benefit ICT-powered global radiation oncology, but also healthcare in general and socio-economic development. This will provide opportunities for healthcare and businesses to grow on the internet. At the Harvard GHC cancer summit, Charles Ayo, the Vice-Chancellor of Covenant University in Nigeria, highlighted other areas that are already emerging in Nigeria and would benefit from greater investment in broadband: eGovernment/eDemocracy; ePolicing, eHealth and eLearning, amongst others.

2.8 Cultural challenges

When collaborating internationally, participants bring unique cultural perspectives and expectations to a project. While such differences are often productive and enriching, they may also present challenges, with a higher risk of misunderstandings that can even slow down a project. Some analyses show that the best science comes from international collaborations [24]. However, collaborators need to be culturally aware and sensitive. This is not only true for research and education efforts, but also for clinical care and investments. In fact, with the field of radiation oncology global health growing, and more investments being made in LMIC to close the cancer divide, there will be an increasing need and more opportunities to address cultural issues, along with ethical and social issues, in global health. Including diaspora healthcare professionals in global health collaborations could help assuage some of these cultural issues, since diaspora members have the greatest appreciation of both partnering countries' cultures. Hence, there may be added justification or opportunity here to engage the diaspora more.

2.9 Access

Even if there is radiotherapy infrastructure and capacity, many in LMIC may still not be able to access cancer care due to cost issues or lack of universal health coverage (UHC). Despite progress in the fight against lethal global diseases such as HIV/AIDS, malaria and other infectious diseases, each year the number of people falling into poverty due to the cost of medical care is growing. It is estimated that each year around 100 million people fall into poverty because of illnesses, and that around one billion people cannot even access the health care they need, paving the way for the spread of disease outbreaks around the globe and a vicious cycle of poverty, disease and threats to global health security. UHC means that all people have access to the health services they need without the risk of financial hardship when paying for them. Essential health services include treatment for HIV, tuberculosis, malaria, non-communicable diseases and mental health, sexual and reproductive health and child health.

To stress the importance of UHC, the first-ever universal Health Coverage Day was launched on 12 December 2014, an effort sponsored by a global coalition whose members include the Rockefeller Foundation, WHO, the World Bank and more than 500 organizations from around the globe. UHC is crucial for saving lives, ending extreme poverty, building resilience against the health effects of climate change and ending deadly epidemics such as Ebola. Addressing the problem/lack of UHC is also an important investment in human capital, which is necessary for economic growth and development, as elaborated by Harvard Nobel prize-winning economist Amartya Sen. UHC is clearly an important issue to address in the next frontier of global health challenges, i.e. non-communicable diseases like cancer (e.g. cervical cancer), which often follow HIV/AIDs survival.

At the Harvard Summit in 2015, a pioneering UHC scheme was proposed, powered by the resource-laden diaspora and ICTs (telemedicine), and this is currently being developed along with other efforts that could help strengthen health care systems in LMIC.

2.10 Partnership challenges

Partnership building is a key tenet of global radiation oncology (see chapter 4). Partnerships are neither rigid nor static, but fluid and dynamic relationships, which often evolve with time. Because partnerships between developed countries and LMIC will evolve, building capacity and structures that ensure partners are accountable to each other while addressing the needs of their respective stakeholder groups is imperative. Some inherent barriers to effective partnerships include inequality/power imbalances between partners, partners' internal management systems and commitment.

These barriers can be overcome in various ways, including the transfer of responsibility and ownership to the less powerful partner, ensuring that there is trust, equality and mutual understanding, and investment in the necessary internal systems to provide effective support and commitment to the partnership. Such commitments are important for sustainability. The ICEC [16] promotes an approach with the underlying premise that the provision of long-term sustainable progress requires personal commitment. This in turn requires fundamental changes to what is rewarded in one's career and a change to the value system of health care, so that human service is valued along with research, education and clinical care. Sustainability is enhanced by the ability to have a committed percentage of time and a career path with metrics for evaluation and promotion, which is an area where global radiation oncology needs to grow.

Table 2.1 summarizes the common challenges faced in global oncology, together with possible solutions. The challenges, solutions and opportunities described in this chapter are clearly not exhaustive, but provide a useful reference for further efforts as the field of global radiation oncology grows.

A recent article by Burkeen *et al* [25] highlighted a number of programs that offer opportunities to become involved in global health initiatives in radiation oncology in a growing effort to address the different challenges. Some of these programs are highlighted in table 2.2.

Table 2.1. Summary of common challenges faced in global radiation oncology and possible solutions.

Challenges	Some suggested solutions
Dearth or lack of infrastructure	• Establish more infrastructure (see *Lancet* Commission report) [6] • Build on already established infrastructure, e.g. from HIV/AIDs for cervical cancer • Support development of innovative lower-cost technologies • Encourage investment
Perception, stigma, treatment abandonment and patients seeking alternative care in the form of traditional healers	• Provide aggressive education for patients, their families and communities • Provide universal health care coverage
Funding /finance	• Develop/incorporate innovative financing mechanisms • Encourage applications to local foundations and other funding agencies
Human resource shortage	• Increased capacity building, including innovative approaches like e-learning • Retraining and training the trainer for sustainability • Pool human resources, e.g. with the use of ICTs in e-learning with multiple instructors using the available time they have • Encourage partnerships • Engage the diaspora to turn the brain drain into a gain
Access to treatment	• Provide universal health care coverage • Build more infrastructure and encourage investment
Culture	• Training/education • Patience, tolerance and respect • Including the diaspora in collaborations with their original countries
Bandwidth for use of ICTs	• Greater investment in broadband • Development of innovative mHealth or ICTpowered apps for LMIC
Space–time	• Use of ICTs • Establish a career progression path for global radiation oncology • Encourage regional collaborations

Table 2.1. (Continued.)

Challenges	Some suggested solutions
No career progression path/commitment	• Establish a career progression path for global radiation oncology • Involve high-level institutional administrators when developing partnerships

Table 2.2. Some global radiation oncology opportunities.

Opportunities	Description
ASTRO/ARRO Global Health Scholars program	This program is designed to enable residents to develop a greater appreciation for the culture and attitudes related to cancer care, with the goal of creating a global perspective on oncology and treatment in LMIC.Association of Residents in Radiation Oncology. Global Health Initiative. Available at: www.astro.org/ARRO/Global-Health-Initiative/Index.aspx
ASCO Health Volunteers Overseas program	This program aims to recruit oncology physicians, including faculty and residents in their final year, who can share their medical expertise and build sustainable relationships with physicians associated with cancer centers in LMIC. American Society of Clinical Oncologists. ASCO International Programs. Available at: www.asco.org/international-programs
IAEA internship program	This program provides medical students and residents with the chance to gain practical work experience and exposes them to the work of the IAEA and the United Nations as a whole. International Atomic Energy Agency. Internship Program. Available at: www.iaea.org/About/Jobs/internships.html
Radiating Hope	Radiating Hope offers medical students and residents the opportunity to participate in such projects as Cancer Care, which provides basic hygiene items to cancer patients and hospitals, and the Senegal Project, in which members help update the Cancer Center in Senegal. Available at: www.radiatinghope.org/get-involved/
Seed Global Health	Supports volunteer physicians and nurses as faculty for one-year rotations in medical and nursing schools in Malawi, Tanzania, Uganda and Swaziland (nursing opportunities only) to address this persistent shortage of health care professionals. Available at: http://seedglobalhealth.org/apply/#.VqQIgOlZVUQ

References

[1] www.southafrica.org.tr/index.php?option=com_content&view=article&id=129%3Ait-always-seems-impossible-until-its-done-nelson-mandela&catid=36%3Asouth-africa-turkish-news&Itemid=64&lang=en

[2] Ngwa W *et al* 2016 *Closing the Cancer Divide through Ubuntu: Information and Communication Technology Powered Models for Global Radiation Oncology* at press
[3] Kate K 2012 Insight: cancer in Africa: fighting a nameless enemy *Reuters*
[4] Denise G 2013 The cancer divide: Uganda fights stigma and poverty to take on breast cancer *New York Times*
[5] 2016 From particle physics, to radiation oncology, to health http://berkeleysciencereview.com/from-particle-physics-to-radiation-oncology-to-public-health/ Accessed, January 10, 2016
[6] Atun R *et al* 2015 Expanding global access to radiotherapy *Lancet Oncol.* **16** 1153–86
[7] Petereit D G and Coleman C N 2015 Editorial: global challenges in radiation oncology *Front. Oncol.* **5** 103
[8] Zubizarreta E H, Fidarova E, Healy B and Rosenblatt E 2015 Need for radiotherapy in low and middle income countries—the silent crisis continues *Clin. Oncol. (R. Coll. Radiol.)* **27** 107–14
[9] Abdel-Wahab M, Bourque J M, Pynda Y, Izewska J, Van der Merwe D, Zubizarreta E and Rosenblatt E 2013 Status of radiotherapy resources in Africa: an International Atomic Energy Agency analysis *Lancet Oncol.* **14** e168–175
[10] Datta N R, Samiei M and Bodis S 2014 Radiation therapy infrastructure and human resources in low- and middle-income countries: present status and projections for 2020 *Int. J. Radiat. Oncol. Biol. Phys.* **89** 448–57
[11] Rosenblatt E, Zubizarreta E, Wondergem J, Fidarova E and Izewska J 2012 The International Atomic Energy Agency (IAEA): an active role in the global fight against cancer *Radiother. Oncol.* **104** 269–71
[12] Datta N R, Samiei M and Bodis S 2014 Radiation therapy infrastructure and human resources in low- and middle-income countries: present status and projections for 2020. In reply to Sharma *et al Int. J. Radiat. Oncol. Biol. Phys.* **90** 971–2
[13] Datta N R, Samiei M and Bodis S 2015 Are state-sponsored new radiation therapy facilities economically viable in low- and middle-income countries? *Int. J. Radiat. Oncol. Biol. Phys.* **93** 229–40
[14] Adewole I *et al* 2014 Building capacity for sustainable research programmes for cancer in Africa *Nat. Rev Clin. Oncol.* **11** 251–9
[15] http://grants.nih.gov/grants/guide/rfa-files/RFA-CA-15-001.html
[16] Coleman C N *et al* 2014 The international cancer expert corps: a unique approach for sustainable cancer care in low and lower-middle income countries *Front. Oncol.* **4** 333
[17] Murray C J, Anderson B, Burstein R, Leach-Kemon K, Schneider M, Tardif A and Zhang R 2011 Development assistance for health: trends and prospects *Lancet* **378** 8–10
[18] Lu C, Mejia-Guevara I, Hill K, Farmer P, Subramanian S V and Binagwaho A 2016 Community-based health financing and child stunting in rural Rwanda *Am. J. Public Health* **106** 49–55
[19] Binagwaho A, Wagner C M and Farmer P E 2016 A vision for global cancer medicine: pursuing the equity of chance *J. Clin. Oncol.* **34** 3–5
[20] www.who.int/tobacco/economics/innovative_financing/en/
[21] http://apps.who.int/iris/bitstream/10665/44371/1/9789241564021_eng.pdf
[22] Mullan F and Kerry V B 2014 The global health service partnership: teaching for the world *Acad. Med.* **89** 1146–8

[23] Ngwa W *et al* 2015 Potential for information and communication technologies to catalyze global collaborations in radiation oncology *Int. J. Radiat. Oncol. Biol. Phys.* **91** 444–7
[24] Adams J 2013 Collaborations: the fourth age of research *Nature* **497** 557–60
[25] Burkeen J, Coleman C N, Daphtary M and Vikram B 2014 The medical student perspective on global health care in radiation oncology: opportunities, barriers to sustainability, and future directions *Int. J. Radiat. Oncol. Biol. Phys.* **89** 492–4

Chapter 3

Current models of global radiation oncology

If you want to go fast, go alone. If you want to go far, go together.
African proverb

3.1 The twinning partnership model for global radiation oncology

3.1.1 Anatomy of twinning partnerships

Twinning partnerships are one of the key emerging models for global radiation oncology, as seen in examples where developed world institutions 'adopt' institutions in LMIC [1]. According to WHO, partnership in this context is a collaborative relationship between two or more parties based on trust, equality and mutual understanding for the achievement of a specified goal. International twinning partnerships intrinsically involve partnerships between two departments/institutions. Successful twinning partnerships usually include the following key features.

1. *Human resources.* People from both sides are needed as the key resource in partnerships. In this case they have the common goals of making radiotherapy services available to patients and advancing cancer research and education.
2. *Commitment.* The partners in the twinning program need a long-term commitment, with twinning programs usually evolving into mutually beneficial long-term partnerships which may grow from one area, e.g. cancer care, into other areas like research and education collaborations. Commitment was listed by global health leaders as one of the challenges for global radiation oncology during the Harvard GHC cancer summit in 2015, emphasizing its importance.
3. *Funding.* Sustained funding is vital for any successful twinning partnership. This may require financial support from diverse public and private sources. It may begin with seed funding from one or more of the partnering institutions

doi:10.1088/978-0-7503-1224-0ch3

as a show of commitment, followed by external funding for longer-term collaborations.

4. *Planning and vision.* A vision is needed for any long-term partnership. Planning for the long term to realize this vision is crucial for success. Such planning is also helpful for securing the required funding, program assessment and adjustments of strategies and deeds as the partnership evolves over time.
5. *Knowledge sharing.* Knowledge sharing/transfer is a vital part of developing successful sustainable partnerships. Aggregating data and experiences, pooling knowledge and learning from each other nourishes the partnership. Knowledge sharing with a clearly defined and progressively implemented policy of evidence-based practice is actually needed as part of planning. Sharing or dissemination of outcomes from program evaluation can also help facilitate progress, and the securing of further funding for sustainability. Knowledge sharing should in general allow for access to timely and accurate information.
6. *Community awareness and participation.* Professor Paul Farmer from Harvard University, who is widely regarded as a global health pioneer, has touted the importance of involving the community in combating diseases. The challenge in global health, he says, is to combat perceptions that health problems are insurmountable and to build systems that can deliver affordable, commonsense care to poor populations. Through his work with Partners in Health in Haiti and Rwanda, Farmer has demonstrated the benefits of this approach, which can also be adapted to cancer and, in particular, global radiation oncology. Community involvement needs to be addressed early in the twinning program to help with community awareness/education, early diagnosis and mitigation of treatment abandonment. Ngwa *et al* [2] recently emphasized the benefits of also engaging diaspora communities, who understand the cultures of both of the countries (developed and LMIC) in which the partnering institutions are based.
7. *Accountability.* In general, partnerships usually involve both risks and benefits, making shared accountability critical. This also applies to twinning partnerships. The Overseas Development Institute [3] posits that accountability is required at three levels: accountability of partners to their own stakeholders; accountability of partners to each other; and accountability of the partnership to its stakeholders. To ensure accountability, program activities need to be regularly audited/evaluated and reports shared with partners and stakeholders. The core dimensions for accountability include transparency, participation, evaluation, and complaints and their redress. Effective accountability also requires partners to understand their responsibilities and rights and embodies trust in each order to act accordingly.

Based on the examination of successful twinning partnerships such as those of St Jude's Hospital with different LMIC, it can be observed that there are a number

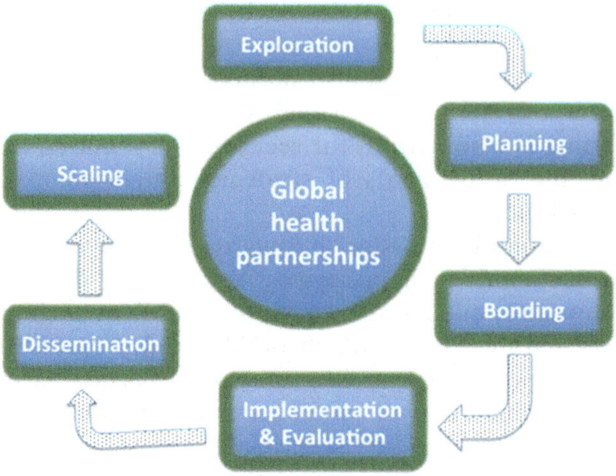

Figure 3.1. Partnership process flow chart.

of phases in a twinning partnership, as represented in the flow chart in figure 3.1. Obviously, some phases may not be equally relevant for every partnership, but they are all included here to serve as a guide.

Exploration (needs assessment) phase

The first important phase of establishing a twinning partnership is the exploration phase, which includes an initial assessment of the specific gaps that need to be addressed and the ability of partners to work together in addressing the identified gaps, taking into account environmental factors at the potential twinning partner institutions. Some of the key requirements that may need to be fulfilled during the exploratory phase include the following.

- Identifying leaders from both organizations, e.g. medical physicists, radiation oncologists, radiation therapists and nurses, who will oversee and coordinate all twinning activities.
- Securing the support of senior leadership, at least at the department level. Such support could include financial or human resources, with a dedicated effort needed to get the program going.
- Ensuring the availability of the minimum required facilities and resources needed to launch the partnership.
- Completing a strength, weakness, opportunity, threat (SWOT) analysis that can be used to guide the partners. This can be very helpful in establishing the vision of the partnership and the strategic plan. To this end, site visits by representatives from the partnering parties are highly recommended, during which initial site surveys can be conducted as part of the SWOT. The SWOT analysis may serve as a benchmark for evaluating current conditions and developing a comprehensive five-year plan.

Planning phase

The outcomes of the exploratory phase allow the establishment of a partnership vision and common overall goal or specific aims that can be used for planning. The establishment of an initial five-year strategic plan is highly recommended in the development of a twinning partnership, or any partnership, for that matter. A comprehensive, strategically focused plan is essential for the successful execution of any partnership and serves as a roadmap to guide the parties. In general, planning should include:

- a vision and overall goal for the partnership or mission statement;
- specific aims or objectives, with measurable outcomes;
- a strategic plan for community engagement;
- an analysis of costs and benefits;
- contingency plans that take potential challenges into account, including those highlighted in chapter 2 in the case of global radiation oncology;
- a stakeholder analysis;
- the possible disease focus, with the priority on areas where an impact can be established more quickly during the first five years of the twinning partnership;
- the identification of lead persons at both partner departments/institutions who will be responsible for each goal;
- a timeline for the completion of specific outcomes, expected deliverables and contingency plans;
- an operational budget with the short- and long-term resources required and allocated
- a plan for regular communication amongst partners and stakeholders;
- a sustainable financing/funding plan;
- a plan for program evaluation, including annual reviews with plans to implement contingency planning or adjustments, as needed;
- a plan for knowledge sharing and wide dissemination of project outcomes; this could include plans for regular workshops/summits/conferences and exchange visits to bolster the collaboration;
- a plan for authorship and ethics, intellectual property, responsible conduct of collaboration activities, etc

Bonding phase: partnership establishment

Following the planning phase, a formal partnership agreement can be established. This can range from a memorandum of understanding through to an explicit legal agreement that details the partnership between the parties. The agreement document essentially expresses a convergence of will between the partnering parties, indicating an intended common line of action, and may not imply a legal commitment with the binding power of a contract. Twinning partnerships may have business or financial issues associated with them and written agreements are helpful to ensure that they are addressed and agreed upon to guide the partnership program. Written agreements may also serve as a reference for arbitration or resolution if disagreements arise during the implementation phase. During the bonding phase, partners should be provided with opportunities to learn about the institutions and people involved.

Implementation and evaluation phase

During the implementation phase, partners essentially begin execution of the plan and associated activities, regularly communicating and addressing issues of concern or contingencies that may arise. Partners bond even more by learning from shared experiences, building on what works well and addressing what does not work well. During implementation, partners are fully committed to ensuring accountability as described above, and to achieving positive measurable outcomes.

The implementation phase can also include regular program evaluation and exchange visits.

Exchange visits allow partners to observe the progress being made and the challenges being faced directly, which can further motivate the partnership. Such regular evaluations should lead to documentation of the outcomes and impact of the program, which can help in securing more support.

Dissemination phase

The measurable outcomes, impact and other documented content should be published and widely disseminated. Publications should be shared with all stakeholders and partners appropriately credited. Celebrating successful outcomes and the progress made towards achieving the planned goals or objectives is also encouraged during this phase. Partners can formalize a process to celebrate progress and significant accomplishments, which is important in building and further motivating improved performance and further success. With respect to dissemination, an example of a suitable time for celebration is after an article is accepted for publication in a peer-reviewed journal. Such publications increase the visibility of the collaboration and facilitate the securing of further funding, while also providing a way to engage the news media to further recognize and publicize the initiative.

Scaling phase

After the initial five-year plan has been executed successfully, it may be time to gradually scale the program. This could be done by adding more programs or by supporting replication with other institutions. The successes of the program should be shared, allowing strengths to be built on while any weaknesses are minimized. Such knowledge sharing can also help others entering into the field to replicate or adapt the model.

Examples of global radiation oncology twinning partnerships

Perhaps one salient example of a twinning partnership in global radiation oncology is the BOTSwana Oncology Global Outreach program (BOTSOGO) [4, 5]. After a year-long exploratory phase in 2011, the Massachusetts General Hospital (MGH)/ Harvard Medical School community partnered with the oncology community in Botswana to form BOTSOGO. The stated ultimate goal of this twinning partnership is to improve access to quality cancer care in Botswana by educating the Botswana population, training future generations of cancer caregivers and conducting vital clinical research. This collaboration was built on a previously existing relationship in HIV/AIDS research and care delivery, developed within the Botswana–Harvard AIDS Institute Partnership.

Over the first five years the partnership was organized around (1) on-site visiting to share expertise in clinical cancer care for capacity-building purposes in identified areas of greatest need and (2) regular tumor boards for multidisciplinary case discussion powered by information and communication technologies (WebEx, Santa Clara, CA). The BOTSOGO program helped to develop the brachytherapy program at Gaborone Private Hospital (GPH) by providing hands-on training, practice-changing guidance for treatment planning, equipment selection, ultrasound image guidance, source insertion and patient treatment. The clinical care and capacity-building effort helped the oncologists at GPH to develop significant expertise, leading to the treatment of up to 50 brachytherapy cases per month. The program has grown to include all cancer-related disciplines, with regular site visits. A full-time MGH faculty has been based in Botswana since 2014 to provide specialized clinical care, train medical students and residents, assist with quality improvement measures and conduct research.

The BOTSOGO tumor boards are said to constitute the first sustainable multidisciplinary tumor boards in Botswana, and they connect the Botswana oncology community (including oncologists, surgeons, pathologists, infectious disease physicians, house officers, nurses, therapists and students) with MGH/Harvard-based disease site experts. The tumor boards meet monthly to discuss specific patient management challenges and can be highly educational.

The BOTSOGO program now regularly publishes/disseminates in leading journals, such as the *Red Journal*, the *Oncologist*, the *New England Journal of Medicine*, the *Journal of Clinical Oncology*, etc The collaboration has also conducted an oncology symposium to catalyze the development of a Botswana comprehensive cancer control plan, standardize cancer treatment guidelines, stimulate local engagement in oncology research and improve the provision of cancer care [4].

The BOTSOGO program is just one example of the growing number of twinning partnerships in global radiation oncology. Others include those linking the University of California, San Diego with the Institute Joliot Curie Cancer Center in Dakar [6]; Emory's Department of Radiation Oncology with the former Soviet republic of Georgia [7]; and the Fred Hutchinson Cancer Center with the Uganda Cancer Institute, which led to the construction of the first comprehensive cancer center built jointly by US and African cancer institutions in sub-Saharan Africa [8]. Twinning partnerships established through the IAEA are also helping to improve radiotherapy for common pediatric cancers in different LMIC [9].

All in all, it is clear that twinning partnerships as above can have a tremendous impact in global radiation oncology. Nobel prize laureate Muhammad Yunus showed that the return on an investment can be greater when aid is divided into small parcels and given to motivated individuals who have a personal stake in a project's outcome [1]. This is a major strength of the twinning partnership model, along with the fact that such partnerships are less complex in the implementation phase because they have fewer partners, i.e. essentially two leading partners.

Thanks to the emergence of advanced ICTs such as the internet, a new and exciting form of twinning collaboration between two institutions is now developing, called e-twinning. Using ICTs, collaborators across institutions can enjoy the thrills of international collaboration at a lower cost than for traditional twinning partnerships. E-twinning is a relatively recent concept, but it has already proven its value in some places. The European Commission started an e-twinning initiative in 2004 and now thousands of schools are participating in Europe [10]. Here, in contrast to traditional twinning partnerships, where people have to travel between countries, the e-twinning projects can be implemented at a very low cost, eliminating both travel costs and travel time. In Europe, partners can agree to work with components from e-learning platforms and this can be done by any institution with a few computers, an internet subscription and committed staff and learners. The use of ICTs and emerging low-cost technologies is covered more explicitly in chapters 4 and 5.

3.2 The consortium partnership model

3.2.1 Anatomy of a consortium

Consortium literally means 'partnership' or 'association' in Latin. A consortium has a more-or-less similar anatomy to a twinning partnership, with the main difference being that consortia usually refer to partnerships involving more than two parties. Like a twinning partnership, a consortium usually also has a common goal. A loose consortium is characterized by an informal partnership arrangement between different parties, where all parties agree to work together to common aims and there may or may not be a written partnership agreement and/or a steering group. Such consortia are fairly easy to set up, with minimal costs, and can build on the strengths of partners, while providing opportunities to share learning, knowledge, good practice, etc. The drawback of a loose consortium is that this model does not offer joint bargaining power.

More structured consortia typically have some form of leadership or steering committee structure, with representatives from each of the parties. However, a consortium can still have no separate legal status. A consortium agreement is usually also put into place among the different parties, which explicitly sets out their legal rights and obligations. One of the parties could be designated the lead organization, which applies for funding on behalf of consortium members, manages the contract and distributes funds to other members via sub-contracting arrangements for particular services or outputs. Usually the lead organization would be the one with the most established reputation, who might be perceived as less 'risky' by funders. However, because there are more entities to manage, it can be difficult to establish a clear identity and 'brand' for a consortium, and more investment is required to establish some level of trust and integration. Consequently, consortia may take more time to develop. All the same, once established, a consortium may be able to leverage the complementary strengths of the partnering parties to be more impactful.

A consortium example in global radiation oncology

One example of an established global radiation oncology consortium is paRTner. paRTner is a partnership for radiotherapy that was started in 2011 by the Department of Medical Physics and Bioengineering at University College London (UCL) in collaboration with the radiotherapy departments of University College London Hospitals and the Royal Berkshire NHS Foundation Trust. The partner institutions in Ghana are the Korle-Bu Teaching Hospital (KBTH), Accra, and Komfo Anokye Teaching Hospital (KATH), Kumasi. The partnership was formed with the goal of supporting Ghana's transition to LINAC technology [11]. In paRTner, the European partners offer hands-on training in conjunction with the development of distance-learning tools, and visit to help commission the LINACs and introduce the first quality system in Ghana. The program also partners Ghanaian radiotherapy medical physics and engineering staff with United Kingdom counterparts who can assist remotely with equipment faults and plan complex LINAC treatments. Another objective is to establish an engineering program for preventative maintenance that would allow up to 700 additional patients to receive treatment per year.

Another example of a noteworthy consortium with a radiation oncology component is the Academic Model for Providing Access to Healthcare (AMPATH) [12]. This consortium, led by the Indiana University School of Medicine in the USA, also includes the Moi University School of Medicine and the Moi Teaching and Referral Hospital (MTRH) in Kenya, the Alpert Medical School of Brown University, Purdue University, the Hubert Yeargan Center for Global Health at Duke University Medical Center, the University of Massachusetts Medical School, the Lehigh Valley Health Network of Pennsylvania, the Eck Institute for Global Health at Notre Dame University, Providence Portland Medical Center and the University of Utah School of Medicine in the USA, and the University of Toronto Faculty of Medicine in Canada. The consortium also partners with the government of Kenya. The partnership has grown since 2001, when it opened its first clinics, with cancer now being only one of the many disease areas it has scaled to address. The AMPATH consortium partner institutions engage in student and faculty exchange, clinical care, training and research, all essential for successfully addressing the short- and long-term challenges of global health. AMPATH's developing Center of Excellence in Cancer Care, called the AMPATH Oncology Institute (AOI), aims to be the premier cancer program in sub-Saharan Africa, with excellence in cancer research, prevention, treatment and palliative care. AMPATH has also partnered with the United States Agency for International Development (USAID) and Pfizer [13].

Ultimately, this consortium partnership aims to develop a sustainable and comprehensive academic clinical care program that will serve Kenyan citizens. To this end, education/training and research are important thrusts of the partnership. Besides building capacity for clinical care, education and training establish a solid foundation upon which important research questions can be investigated. The AOI initiative also, amongst other activities, organizes grant-writing workshops as part of its training to build up research capacity. Cognizant of the importance of community engagement, all of AMPATH's programs are designed to involve Kenyans. AMPATH has also integrated the use of ICTs, as evidenced by the use of an advanced electronic medical record system to enable cost savings through task-shifting in clinical care. It is reported that over 100 sites globally now host the AMPATH-originated Open Medical Records System, OpenMRS [13]. The program is also working closely with the Kenyan Ministry of Health on developing an income security program for patients, so they are able to pay for the care they receive.

3.3 The non-profit model for global radiation oncology

3.3.1 Anatomy of the non-profit model

Non-profit organizations with the express mission to support global radiation oncology are essentially structured as typical non-profit organizations. They use any surplus revenues to further achieve their purpose or mission, rather than distributing the surplus income to the organization's stakeholders as profit or dividends. Such non-profit organizations can take the form of a corporation, an individual enterprise (e.g., individual charitable contributions), an unincorporated association, or a foundation. For global radiation oncology, non-profit organizations may also include academic institutions, public charities, public clinics and hospitals, legal aid societies, volunteer services organizations, professional associations, research institutes and even governmental agencies. Because non-profit organizations are usually registered in states, they would have to be registered separately in other countries in order to operate there as independent entities. Because they can also be involved in twinning or consortium partnerships, the category focus here is on non-profit organizations that support global radiation oncology activity, but are not necessarily directly involved in a partnership with another entity.

Examples of global radiation oncology non-profit organizations

One example of non-profit organization with a mission that has a significant focus on global radiation oncology is Radiating Hope [6, 14]. Its goal is to update and provide radiation equipment to developing countries and to advance cancer care in those countries. Radiating Hope is one hundred per cent volunteer-run and has the following specific goals:

- improve cancer care, specifically radiation oncology care, around the globe;
- deliver radiation equipment to countries where oncologic care is limited;
- assist with effective, safe and sustainable use of equipment;
- provide intensive in-person and remote training long term;
- raise funds and awareness;
- forge partnerships between medical professionals and equipment manufacturers;
- educate and empower local communities and institutions through formal partnerships with US institutions and physicians.

As part of its activities to achieve this mission, Radiating Hope organizes medical missions, such as the one to Senegal in 2012, whose primary objective was to provide Senegal with its first high-dose-rate (HDR) brachytherapy afterloader. The HDR afterloader was a private donation via a clinic in New Jersey (USA) and corporate sponsorship from Nucletron (Veenendaal, the Netherlands). Others have also donated brachytherapy devices, equipment, treatment planning software and different supplies. Besides implementing the HDR brachytherapy unit in Senegal, the Radiating Hope team followed this with three training visits for technical support, providing extra in-person training. Furthermore, Radiating Hope team members continued to provide remote weekly quality assurance/technical support and training for staff in Senegal through three Radiating Hope physicists. Training sessions were for PLATO treatment planning and used screen-sharing software. They also provided remote support to help transition Senegal from 2D treatment to 3D conformal radiation therapy. Radiating Hope is also looking to support the establishment of a radiotherapy center in Tanzania and to support other developing countries, in line with its mission.

Other radiation oncology non-profit organizations are also emerging, including: ICEC [15], Medical Physics Without Borders (MPWB) [2], MEPHIDA and Treatsafely [16], amongst others. While long-term partnerships are desirable, in global health, some activity supported by non-profit organizations may be temporary, but with longer-term implications. For example, many organizations such as Seed Global Health [17] support 'train the trainer' approaches to build sustainable capacity in LMIC. In this recently trending educational model, an individual or group in need of a skill is teamed up with an entity possessing more expert knowledge. The learning can occur through various mechanisms, face to face or via micro-lectures, usually delivered with the help of the internet and other ICTs. With this modus operandi, knowledge can become more democratic and decentralized, furthering a process in which the learning continues, as those who have been trained by the 'expert' quickly transition into resident or regional experts and subsequently train others and disseminate knowledge.

A non-profit at the individual level can simply be a volunteer, who also participates in global health efforts when circumstances allow. Many residents and radiation oncology health professionals have volunteered their time and effort to support global health efforts at the individual level, including during their vacation time. Such individual/volunteer level contributions to global health can be further facilitated through some of the scholarships or funding provided by non-profit organizations who support global health, or via ICTs.

References

[1] Zietman A Bringing 2014 radiation therapy to underserved nations: an increasingly global responsibility in an ever-shrinking world *Int. J. Radiat. Oncol. Biol. Phys.* **89** 440–2

[2] Ngwa W *et al* 2016 *Closing the Cancer Divide through Ubuntu: Information and Communication Technology Powered Models for Global Radiation Oncology* at press

[3] *Partnerships and Accountability: Current Thinking and Approaches Among Agencies Supporting Civil Society Organisations* www.odi.org/sites/odi.org.uk/files/odi-assets/publications-opinion-files/158.pdf Accessed 10 January 2016

[4] Efstathiou J A *et al* 2014 Addressing the growing cancer burden in the wake of the AIDS epidemic in Botswana: the BOTSOGO collaborative partnership *Int. J. Radiat. Oncol. Biol. Phys.* **89** 468–75

[5] Efstathiou J A *et al* 2016 Establishing and delivering quality radiation therapy in resource-constrained settings: the story of Botswana *J. Clin. Oncol.* **34** 27–35

[6] Einck J P *et al* 2014 Implementation of a high-dose-rate brachytherapy program for carcinoma of the cervix in Senegal: a pragmatic model for the developing world *Int. J. Radiat. Oncol. Biol. Phys.* **89** 462–7

[7] Jani A B, Esiashvili N, Cassels D, Godette K and Johnstone P A 2008 International collaborations in radiation oncology: a single-institution experience in academic outreach *J. Am. Coll. Radiol* **5** 1001–6

[8] www.fredhutch.org/en/news/center-news/2015/05/what-Uganda-is-teaching-about-cancer.html Accessed 7 January 2016

[9] Salminen E, Anacak Y, Laskar S, Kortmann R D, Raslawski E, Stevens G and Ribeiro R C 2009 Twinning partnerships through International Atomic Energy Agency (IAEA) to improve radiotherapy in common paediatric cancers in low- and mid-income countries *Radiother. Oncol.* **93** 368–71

[10] www.etwinning.net/en/pub/progress/awards/european_prizes.htm

[11] www.ucl.ac.uk/medphys/international/partner/ghana Accessed 3 January 2016

[12] Moormann A, Skiles J, Koros E, Asirwa F C, Busakhala N and Loehrer P 2013 Mentoring future Kenyan oncology researchers *Infect. Agent Cancer* **8** 40

[13] www.ampathkenya.org/ Accessed 7 January 2016

[14] Fisher B J, Daugherty L C, Einck J P, Suneja G, Shah M M, Dad L K, Mutter R W, Wilkinson J B and Mundt A J 2014 Radiation oncology in Africa: improving access to cancer care on the African continent *Int. J. Radiat. Oncol. Biol. Phys.* **89** 458–61

[15] Coleman C N *et al* 2014 The international cancer expert corps: a unique approach for sustainable cancer care in low and lower-middle income countries *Front. Oncol.* **4** 333

[16] https://i.treatsafely.org/ Accessed 3 January 2016

[17] Mullan F and Kerry V B 2014 The global health service partnership: teaching for the world *Acad. Med.* **89** 1146–8

Chapter 4

ICT-powered models of global radiation oncology

Information and communications technology (ICT) are indispensable to global health.

Fogarty International [1]

4.1 Potential of ICTs to catalyze global radiation oncology

Recently, Ngwa *et al* highlighted the potential of ICTs to catalyze high-impact international collaborations in radiation oncology care, research and education [2–4]. ICTs refer to devices or systems that allow the storage, retrieval, manipulation, transmission and receipt of digital/electronic information. Examples include smartphones, personal computers, digital television, e-mail, social media platforms, radio, Skype, etc. In context of the challenges of making radiotherapy accessible in LMIC, ICTs present enormous opportunities for facilitating activities that can have a significant impact right away, making ongoing global radiation oncology initiatives more effective and converting the recent upsurge of global health interest into greater concerted action, and working towards improved health outcomes, saved lives and the elimination of worldwide cancer disparities. Some examples of ICTs that can be employed to catalyze global health collaborations are shown in table 4.1.

Following the AAPM 2014 symposium on the potential of ICTs to catalyze global health collaborations in radiation oncology, the GHC program at the Dana Farber/Harvard Cancer Center was initiated, with its primary focus being on catalyzing global radiation oncology by leveraging ICTs, with this complemented by unprecedented outreach to industry, the diaspora, etc. The program recognized that many people want to participate in global health, but are limited by the space–time travel requirements, in addition to the financial constraints. Using ICTs, many

doi:10.1088/978-0-7503-1224-0ch4

Table 4.1. Examples of ICTs or ICTs platforms for global radiation oncology.

Examples of ICTs and ICT-powered activities to catalyze radiation oncology (RadOnc) global health collaborations	Potential uses
Care	
Video conferencing ICTs, e.g. Adobe Connect, Cisco WebEx, Citrix GoToMeeting, Microsoft Lync, Skype, Google Hangouts, etc	Facilitate remote consultations and tumor boards
Remote treatment planning ICTs: e.g. Varian VelocityGrid, Elekta MOSAIQ and Nucletron PLATO treatment planning using screen-sharing software	Facilitate space–time flexible remote support in treatment planning, quality assurance and evaluation
GHC-supported mHealth Apps, FaceTime, Google Glass, etc	Facilitate remote support, e.g. for machine QA and maintenance
Research	
ICT software (e.g., Profiles, SHRINE and eagle-i)	Provide enhanced ability to find each other and form teams: complementary collaborators/mentors across institutions in different countries
Computational Environment for Radiotherapy Research (CERR)	Pronounced 'sir', this is a software platform for developing and sharing research results in radiation therapy treatment planning
Microsoft Cloud, with Microsoft Azure, Windows Server and Microsoft System Center	Cloud computing and big data research collaborations
Education/training	
EdX, CourseSites, VUCCnet	For e-learning with learning modules, multimedia and facilitating more space–time flexible participation in teaching/learning
Chartrounds.com platform	Continuous education
Multimedia library, tablet computers with educational content: books, task group reports, archived lectures, etc	Enhanced access to electronic education materials, practice guidelines and journal articles; extended lectures beyond the classroom

people who might not be able to travel can still participate in and contribute to global health, as in the examples shown in table 4.1. With ICTs, literally anyone, from students through faculty to retirees, can participate in cancer care, research or education. In cancer care, for example, radiation oncologists and other cancer care team members can work together securely on a patient's treatment planning, evaluation and delivery across institutions using currently available treatment planning software like Varian's VelocityGrid, Elekta's MOSAIQ and so forth. In addition, advanced ICTs like Google Glass, FaceTime and Skype can be used for remote support of radiotherapy machine quality assurance (QA) and lower cost maintenance to minimize machine downtime, which is a major issue for many LMIC.

In research, advances in ICTs such as WebEx (video-conferencing software) can be employed to enable remote participation at conferences, providing opportunities for greater interaction to begin or for existing scientific collaborations to be nurtured. A 2014 Nigeria Prostate Cancer Conference provides an example of this: US radiation oncology faculty, who could not travel because of the Ebola virus, still successfully participated via WebEx, which was much appreciated by the local Nigerian participants. Cloud computing platforms can also facilitate global radiation oncology research collaborations. In 2015, ASTRO, the National Cancer Institute and the AAPM co-sponsored a two-day workshop for radiation oncology physicians and physicists, focused on opportunities for radiation oncology in the era of big data. The Big Data Workshop highlighted opportunities for radiation oncology in big data research, such as current big data cancer registries, safety and incident reporting systems and other strategies that will have the greatest impact on radiation oncology research, quality assurance, safety and outcomes analysis. Another example where such collaborations are readily feasible is in the emerging field of radiomics [5–8]. Here, radiomics refers to the extraction and analysis of large quantities of advanced quantitative imaging features with high throughput from medical images obtained with computed tomography (CT), positron emission tomography (PET) or magnetic resonance imaging (MRI). Importantly, these data are usually extracted from clinical standard-of-care images, which could result in a very large potential subject pool.

In education, online learning platforms could allow even modest education and training contributions to be made, e.g. from retired faculty teaching a course module for an hour a week, transferring vital knowledge to LMIC trainees to help build capacity. Over 89% of residents surveyed recently [9] indicated a positive interest in participating in global health; their participation in tumor boards powered by ICTs like Adobe Connect could broaden their training or perspective, preparing them to be the next generation of global health leaders. These are just a few examples of potential applications.

4.2 Emerging ICT powered models

Table 4.2 some of the emerging models for ICT-powered radiation oncology collaborations, along with links or references for more information. For simplicity, these models are divided into three main categories: care, research and education. However, some of these model programs may include activities that go beyond just one category. Under cancer care, these include: BOTSOGO [10], Chartrounds.com, the Quality Assurance Review Center (QARC), Cure4Kids and Radiating Hope [11]. Under education, these include: the IAEA Virtual University for Cancer Control (IAEA VUCCnet), the AAPM, the ASTRO and TreatSafely. In research, these include: QARC, the University of Massachusetts Lowell (UML) Medical Physics Program and others.

Table 4.2. Model programs in global radiation oncology powered by ICTs.

Model programs	ICT-powered activities
Care	
BOTSOGO [16] (www.botsogo.org)	Monthly tumor boards and remote support for radiation oncology care
Chartrounds.com (www.chartrounds.com)	Chartrounds brings together academic disease site specialists from leading cancer treatment institutions and connects them with the Chartrounds network of over 1300 physicians and medical physicists. On a scheduled basis, they discuss patient management and treatment plans with trusted colleagues in real time
Cure4kids (www.cure4kids.org)	Cure4Kids is an online resource for healthcare professionals dedicated to enhancing the care of children who have cancer and other life-threatening diseases in countries around the globe
QARC (www.qarc.org)	Provides radiation therapy QA services. Has potential for facilitating international 'chart rounds', maintaining a registry of patients discussed, connecting radiation oncologists with questions about patient treatment to experts in the field using web-based technology and facilitating design of appropriate protocols
Radiating Hope, [17] (http://www.radiatinghope.org/)	Remote treatment planning using screen-sharing software; remote QA and technical support via Brainlab's Quentry system. Remote discussion of difficult cases, contouring and treatment planning
Education	
IAEA PACT VUCCnet (http://cancer.iaea.org)	Online training of RT technicians, cancer prevention community health workers, screening workers, pathologists and pathology technicians, oncology surgeons, palliative care practitioners and data collectors
Cure4kids (www.cure4kids.org)	Cure4Kids offers online education and collaboration tools that are freely available to registered users
Radiating Hope [17] (www.radiatinghope.org)	Remote training of residents and staff in Africa, including on PLATO; data sharing
ASTRO International Education Subcommittee [19]	Oversees ASTRO's international education efforts, with initiatives including: coordination of educational efforts with regional societies including ALATRO, SEAROG, CSTRO, TASTRO, AROI and others. Focus on integrating advanced technologies in LMIC. Remote learning initiatives such as e-contouring on a web-based platform. Support of ARRO for a 3DCRT online learning curriculum for breast cancer and lymphoma and gyn tumors (in upcoming ALATRO conference). Development of educational courses in Spanish and Mandarin at the ASTRO annual meeting

Table 4.2. (Continued.)

Model programs	ICT-powered activities
AAPM (www.aapm.org)	International Education Committee, AAPM online learning center, virtual education library with over 155 educational resources for developing countries, with continuous education credit for medical physicists
drkarenwinkfield.com	Leveraging ICTs to improve access for medically underserved communities in Boston: radio; online courses; audience participation: suitcase radio station; crank radio; digital satellite radio; etc
Global RT (http://globalrt.org)	Provides a virtual platform for education, exchange and action around the essential nature of radiotherapy for cancer care
Research	
QARC (www.qarc.org)	Remote review in support of cancer clinical trials; potentially connecting arrays to appropriate research databases
UMASS Lowell	Remote mentorship of medical physics graduate students with weekly Skype meetings to evaluate progress and guide students
Global Oncology (http://globalonc.org/Projects/global-cancer-project-map)	The Global Cancer Project Map (GCPM): provide resources to view and better understand international efforts in cancer research

4.2.1 Cancer care

The tumor boards from the BOTSOGO model initiative highlighted in table 4.2 represent an excellent ICT-powered approach to enhancing cancer care collaborations. They are also particularly attractive in view of the relatively low cost of setting up the infrastructure for ICT-powered international tumor boards. The impact here includes improvements to the quality of patient care and saved lives. For many LMIC institutions, this could be transformative, promoting a multidisciplinary approach to care and breaking the culture of silos, which many young doctors in LMIC have lamented. In many LMIC healthcare institutions, where resources are scarce and support systems largely unavailable, younger professionals often face daunting challenges, but seeking a second opinion from senior colleagues is viewed as a weakness. The experience from tumor boards also shows that this could be one way to introduce global health to residents, who, arguably, can learn a great deal in real time from LMIC healthcare professionals who manage patients with limited resources. It can certainly help to concretize some of the valuable, but more historical, lower-cost techniques that are learned but rarely used in more developed countries. As indicated previously, most residents surveyed recently expressed an interest in participating in global radiation oncology experiences during their residency training [9]. A growing number of institutions are already conducting regular tumor boards with African LMIC, such as the Fred Hutchinson Cancer Center, Seattle with the Uganda Cancer Institute, Kampala. Furthermore, institutions in East Africa and Dana Farber/Harvard Cancer Center institutions are working to scale this model. Other institutions are being encouraged to do same, because these are potential win–win areas in which to begin global radiation oncology partnerships with a relatively low-cost investment. Moreover, this model can lead to a mutually beneficial impact on patient care while providing valuable experience for residents and other cancer care professionals.

Other areas with major promise and enthusiasm for scale-up include remote support, treatment planning and quality assurance, following the model of Radiating Hope and the QARC (table 4.2). Many institutions in Africa have expressed an interest in this model and are in need of partners. Some have indicated that this would also benefit their residency training programs. Chartrounds.com (table 4.2) is a HIPPA compliant, secure web-based conferencing project that offers radiation oncology health professionals a scheduled one-hour live case review session over the internet with disease-specific specialists in radiation oncology. Through ICT capabilities, Chartrounds has bridged the knowledge gap between community physicians and specialists, resulting in overall improved patient care and reduced cancer care costs.

Because late stage presentation is a serious problem in Africa, such that even if these patients were airlifted to the best cancer centers in the USA and Europe the treatment results would not be any better, a research project was conducted by AORTIC to test whether cancer can be downstaged there by simple educational means and ICT, making it more effectively treatable. In the first year of the project, covering April 2009 to March 2010, stages 1 and 2 made up 23.8% of the 109 cancers diagnosed in the intervention village, while in the control village stages 1 and 2 made up 11.1% of the 36 cancers diagnosed.

In the second year of the project, covering April 2010 to March 2011, stages 1 and 2 made up 50.5% of the 93 cancers diagnosed in the intervention village, while in the control village stages 1 and 2 made up 22.2% of the 18 cancers diagnosed. In the third year of the project, covering April 2011 to March 2012, stages 1 and 2 made up 74.4% of the 43 cancers diagnosed in the intervention villages, while in the control village stages 1 and 2 made up 36.8% of the 19 cancers diagnosed. In summary, this study [12] showed that it is possible to downstage cancer in Africa by simple and affordable educational means and the use of ICTs.

Efforts are ongoing to secure the funding required for scale-up in these areas. Radiating Hope is also working on a model that will pay the salary of western-trained radiation oncology healthcare professionals to lead the development of a Radiating Hope Cancer of Excellence on the African continent. Partnerships with industry and companies who provide radiation oncology technology could be mutually beneficial.

4.2.2 Education/training

There is growing consensus that online education is a powerful paradigm that can significantly complement face-to-face learning where needed. It is also very appealing for many practicing health professionals who work in a clinic and have practical training, but would like to gain graduate instruction towards a master's or doctoral degree or undergo training to conduct research more effectively. Currently, the main structured diploma or online certificate education model in radiation oncology that benefits LMIC institutions directly is the IAEA's VUCCnet (table 4.2). major professional societies, including the ASTRO [13] and the AAPM, have developed online learning content that is tailored to LMIC. ASTRO, within the International Education Subcommittee, has established through its organizational structure a multifaceted forum of volunteers, experts and stakeholders from around the globe to assess educational needs, obstacles and development opportunities in global radiation oncology education. Furthermore, sub-specialty resources are available via Cure4Kids, TreatSafely and other organizations. The GHC program at the Dana Farber/Harvard Cancer Center is now working with faculty at the University of Massachusetts, the MD Anderson Cancer Center, the Health First Cancer Institute, the University of Pennsylvania and the Memorial Sloan Kettering Cancer Center, amongst a growing list of interested partners, to start a structured online learning program delivered via EdX/Coursesites. Other medical physicists are leading efforts to help develop a relevant medical physics curriculum that facilitates both continuous education and the award of a degree or certificate. Funding has been secured for this effort and there is already movement to scale it up in partnership with the IAEA VUCCnet program and the International Organization for Medical Physics (IOMP). The Muhimbili University of Health and Allied Sciences is looking to incorporate various components of ICT-powered radiation oncology education in partnership with others to benefit trainees in the East Africa region.

Recently, ASTRO's Educase e-contouring breast modules were incorporated into a pilot curriculum for the implementation of 3D conformal breast radiation therapy in Armenia [14]. 3D conformal radiation therapy (3DCRT) has been in widespread use in developed nations since the 1990s. By contrast, radiation therapy centers in developing nations are just beginning to adopt this technology. Standardized means for assisting radiation oncologists as they transition from 2D planning to 3DCRT are lacking. The pilot curriculum aims to train radiation oncology professionals in the key processes associated with 3DCRT implementation for breast cancer. Through the online exercises, radiation oncologists practice the proper delineation of tumor target volumes and organs at risk of radiation damage. The utility and feasibility of online learning have been demonstrated through the pilot curriculum and it can be employed at other centers seeking to transition from 2D to 3DCRT, while it can also include other tumor sites. It requires that radiation oncology professionals from both collaborating institutions be both available and flexible. Parallel efforts are ongoing to refine the curriculum and test the intervention in the other collaborating countries.

Education via knowledge sharing through the various volunteers, contributors and stakeholder actors, as exemplified by the 2015 Global Health Catalyst Cancer summit at Harvard [15], will be very useful in advancing global radiation oncology, and global oncology efforts as a whole. Such knowledge sharing should also inform, engage and facilitate the participation of those interested in global health, with *au courant* recommendations on how best to address any challenges or limitations, based on learning from the experience of others. Major national conferences such as those of ASTRO and AAPM now regularly feature sessions on global health, and the *Red Journal* published an extensive series of articles on global health in the past year [16]. It is imperative that leading radiation oncology journals, such as the *Red Journal, Medical Physics*, the *Green Journal* and others, continue to serve as the conscience of this emerging area, by advocating and maintaining awareness of global radiation oncology. Regular meetings such as the GHC summit should also serve as avenues for knowledge sharing, using the experiences of leaders of the different emerging models.

Beyond the radiation oncology community, such knowledge sharing and cancer education can also be carried out via radio, as highlighted by the work of Karen Winkfield, a radiation oncologist who uses this medium to reach minority populations in the Boston area [17]. Such models can be replicated in developing countries, sometimes using suitcase radio stations. Leveraging ICTs such as social media to share evidence-based information and engage in practical discussion would also be a powerful tool for education and sensitization. One organization that is currently implementing this is Radiation Nation (table 4.1), which promotes educational collaborative discussions on radiation oncology that are greatly appreciated in LMIC.

Another possibility is to set up programs to help train LMIC radiation oncologists and other oncology leaders to be more competent in the use of ICTs. Institutions such as the ICT University [18], with growing infrastructure and programs in LMIC, could help in delivering such training. The advantage of the ICT University model is that it allows study to be conducted via its eLearning platform. Covenant University in Nigeria, one of Africa's leading ICT institutions, is also working to become a major hub for facilitating ICT-powered global oncology in West/Central Africa. Members of AORTIC and the Federation of African Medical Physics Organizations have expressed interest in such training and the AORTIC Education and Training Committee is leading a needs assessment effort that can serve as a reference for developing and maximizing its benefits.

Of the estimated 200 000 new cases of children with cancer per year, more than 80% live in LMIC [19]. The real number of children with cancer in many LMIC is not known because of the absence of cancer registries. Cure4Kids (table 4.2) is a model online resource for healthcare professionals dedicated to enhancing the care of children who have cancer and other life-threatening diseases in countries around the globe. Cure4Kids offers online education and collaboration tools for all interested parties. Closing the survival gap through a collective effort using the emerging ICT-powered model is also being assisted by twinning programs, which are particularly effective in pediatric oncology. Developing twinning programs with LMIC is possible and encouraging: it is a modification of the classic example of a partnership of two units from high and low income settings.

4.2.3 Research

ICT-powered models for global radiation oncology research are only beginning to emerge. One is the planned launch of the GHC microgrant competition, referencing the model of the United States National Cancer Institute Beginning Investigator Grant for Catalytic Research (NCI BIG Cat) [20], but incorporating a crowdfunding component. The program will in particular promote transatlantic research collaborations/co-mentorship between LMIC faculty and faculty at National Cancer Institute comprehensive cancer centers such as the Dana Farber/Harvard Cancer Center. A major goal for this effort is to promote the submission of its results in conference abstracts and publications, with co-authors from both LMIC and US institutions. A primary focus is to grow transatlantic partnerships with LMIC in sub-Saharan Africa, help grow visibility for LMIC partners and generate new knowledge or preliminary data that could lead to more grant funding or new hypotheses. The crowdfunding approach [21] will also deliberately grow engagement with the diaspora. It will enhance the appreciation of highly meritorious cancer research that transcends continents, advancing healthcare and economic development.

The development of low-cost technologies in radiation oncology that can be employed and/or maintained easily in LMIC, including mobile health technologies, is also needed, e.g. for treatment, quality assurance, imaging, dosimetry, etc. Some of these technologies continue to be developed, as highlighted at the Harvard summit. The National Cancer Institute currently has a funding mechanism for supporting such research and this should be encouraged for both developed countries and LMIC researchers. Elzawawy recently highlighted some of these resource issues and the associated development of cost-effective radiotherapy techniques and methodologies that would lead to more affordable cancer care for more patients who are in need [22].

4.2.4 Outreach

Complementary outreach that goes beyond what is traditional for radiation oncology has been proposed, e.g. via purposeful engagement/partnerships with the diaspora in global health efforts [21]. For example, many Africans in Diaspora (AiD) feel a strong sense of connection and want to contribute to healthcare and development in their native countries. As an example, even when the recent Ebola crisis was at its peak, the AiD were still travelling to visit their families in Africa when many of the non-Africans heeded the prudent calls of their governments to evacuate. The AiD constitutes one of the most educated diaspora groups in North America, remitting over 40 billion US dollars per year to Africa, which is more than the annual global aid to the continent, while saving another 53 billion US dollars annually [23]. Community outreach involvement of the highly skilled/educated/resourced AiD would undoubtedly spawn and catalyze stronger collaborations and help turn the currently devastating African brain drain into gains against cancer.

Crowdsourcing that employs ICTs is one of the avenues where the AiD can complement global oncology efforts. The diaspora can help address the primary level disparities in cancer education and prevention as well as the stigma associated with cancer in Africa. As Mohammed *et al* showed [24, 25], LMIC citizens are more likely to listen to cancer prevention education and awareness talk from those who share their social fabric and belief systems. The AiD, returning regularly from overseas, may be more effective in this area because of the status they hold in their societies and their greater awareness of both developed country and LMIC cultures. The diaspora can also be crowdsourced for the development of appropriate words for cancer where there is currently a vocabulary deficit, and for the translation of the language of American Cancer Society or National Cancer Institute flyers into appropriate language with a suitable cultural context to better communicate cancer prevention education and awareness in their native LMIC. This was highlighted by Harriet Shangarai, who attended the 2015 Harvard summit with the Tanzanian ambassador to the USA and other Tanzanian diaspora members who were uniting against cancer. Recognizing the significance of communicating about cancer in local languages, and knowledge sharing, Harriet started a Swahili health education blog to benefit her native country of Tanzania and its immigrant population in the USA; to date, this has had over 9000 visitors. This ability to communicate has the potential to alleviate the formidable and unresolved access-to-care challenge through the pathway of cancer prevention. Once diagnosed, those few who can afford therapy may have to trek hundreds of miles to a center with radiotherapy services and then endure enormously long waiting times before receiving care. More than one-third of cancer deaths can be prevented altogether through awareness and early diagnosis. Therefore, given the limited specialty care and radiotherapy services in LMIC, more complementary efforts that can promote cancer prevention are imperative to reduce late diagnosis. This would increase timely access to limited radiotherapy resources and, most importantly, save lives.

Another ICT-powered initiative that is under development and which could strengthen LMIC healthcare systems substantially is partnering with the AiD to develop a pan-African affordable healthcare insurance scheme. The more economically viable diaspora would be encouraged to enroll in this system, with the possibility of extending coverage to their sending country family members, and it would include coverage for cancer care like radiotherapy, support for preventive healthcare, palliative care with provision for basic pain medication, and so on. Such proposals are only a representative sample of the ongoing dialogue with the diaspora.

Another ICT-powered avenue for engaging the diaspora is crowdfunding, mentioned earlier. Given the tens of billions of US dollars in remittances and the additional tens of billions in savings, the diaspora has enormous potential to crowdfund research, in an approach that is growing in popularity in the USA, as seen from the many crowdfunding organizations, e.g. Rockethub, Kickstarter and others. Crowdfunding would be particularly beneficial in resource-poor settings, where even relatively small contributions can lead to many years of fruitful research for cancer researchers who would otherwise have no funding. Such crowdfunding can be used to generate preliminary data to be more competitive when applying for funding, including international funding such as that provided by the US NIH. These preliminary data would also engender new hypotheses for more globally beneficial research and create greater visibility for LMIC researchers working with their developed country peers to publish these data. Cancer research in LMIC will also help in driving public policy, changing perceptions, generating new knowledge and technologies for clinical translation and enabling participation in clinical trials, and it will benefit economic development. Rifat Atun and others are leading global health efforts to highlight the economic/development benefits of investing in closing the cancer divide [26, 27].

ICTs could also help with patient safety. Recent workshops and surveys [28] have highlighted major patient safety issues in the use of radiation technologies in LMIC. When the *New York Times* reported on such incidences in the USA [29] there was a major outcry, leading to testimony in the US Congress by AAPM representatives to address the issue. Imagine the situation where many African countries do not even have a medical physicist, coupled with a dramatic increase in the use of radiation technologies, including for diagnostic imaging. It is crucial to raise public awareness, as the *New York Times* did, and advocate for the recognition of the importance of medical physicists in ensuring the safety of patients, healthcare staff and the general public when using such technologies. The benefits of this will go beyond cancer treatment, as radiation technologies are widely used in diagnostic testing for other diseases, including cardiovascular disease, infectious disease, trauma, musculoskeletal disorders, dentistry, etc. In fact, the absence or shortage of medical physicists in African countries is a silent healthcare crisis, which is likely affecting even policy makers and their family members, even if they are unaware of it. The establishment of an anonymous ICT-powered self-reporting system could be very useful here. This could also then leverage advocacy efforts.

In conclusion, this chapter highlighted the potential of ICTs and emerging ICT-powered approaches to facilitate global radiation oncology collaborations in a variety of ways. Those mentioned are not the only ones that currently exist, but they can provide a useful reference for the expansion of global radiation oncology programs, with scalable activities catalyzed by ICTs and effective outreach.

References

[1] www.fic.nih.gov/NEWS/GLOBALHEALTHMATTERS/Pages/Information-technology.aspx Accessed 3 January 2016

[2] Isabalija S R, Mbarika V and Kituyi G M 2013 A framework for sustainable implementation of e-medicine in transitioning countries *Int. J. Telemed. Appl.* **2013** 615617

[3] Meso P, Mbarika V W and Sood S P 2009 An overview of potential factors for effective telemedicine transfer to sub-Saharan Africa *IEEE Trans. Inf. Technol. Biomed.* **13** 734–9

[4] Pal A, Mbarika V W, Cobb-Payton F, Datta P and McCoy S 2005 Telemedicine diffusion in a developing country: the case of India *IEEE Trans. Inf. Technol. Biomed.* **9** 59–65

[5] Aerts H J *et al* 2014 Decoding tumour phenotype by noninvasive imaging using a quantitative radiomics approach *Nat. Commun.* **5** 4006

[6] Bourgier C, Colinge J, Ailleres N, Fenoglietto P, Brengues M, Pelegrin A and Azria D 2015 Radiomics: definition and clinical development *Cancer Radiother.* **19** 532–7

[7] Cunliffe A, Armato S G, 3rd, Castillo R, Pham N, Guerrero T and Al-Hallaq H A 2015 Lung texture in serial thoracic computed tomography scans: correlation of radiomics-based features with radiation therapy dose and radiation pneumonitis development *Int. J. Radiat. Oncol. Biol. Phys.* **91** 1048–56

[8] Gillies R J, Kinahan P E and Hricak H 2015 Radiomics: images are more than pictures, they are data *Radiology* **2015** 151169

[9] Dad L, Shah M M, Mutter R, Olsen J, Dominello M, Miller S M, Fisher B, Lee N and Komaki R 2014 Why target the globe?: four-year report (2009–2013) of the Association of Residents in Radiation Oncology Global Health Initiative *Int. J. Radiat. Oncol. Biol. Phys.* **89** 485–91

[10] Efstathiou J A 2014 Addressing the growing cancer burden in the wake of the AIDS epidemic in Botswana: the BOTSOGO collaborative partnership *Int. J. Radiat. Oncol. Biol. Phys.* **89** 468–75

[11] Fisher B J, Daugherty L C, Einck J P, Suneja G, Shah M M, Dad L K, Mutter R W, Wilkinson J B and Mundt A J 2014 Radiation oncology in Africa: improving access to cancer care on the African continent *Int. J. Radiat. Oncol. Biol. Phys.* **89** 458–61

[12] Ngoma T and Mandeli, J.F J 2015 Holland downstaging cancer in rural Africa *Int. J. Cancer* **136** 2875–9

[13] Mayr N A 2014 International outreach: what is the responsibility of ASTRO and the major international radiation oncology societies? *Int. J. Radiat. Oncol. Biol. Phys.* **89** 481–4

[14] Ngwa W *et al* 2016 *Closing The Cancer Divide Through Ubuntu: Information and Communication Technology Powered Models for Global Radiation Oncology* at press

[15] GHC 2015 *Global Health Catalyst Events* www.globalhealthcatalystevents.org

[16] Zietman A 2014 Bringing radiation therapy to underserved nations: an increasingly global responsibility in an ever-shrinking world *Int. J. Radiat. Oncol. Biol. Phys.* **89** 440–2

[17] Karen W 2015 www.drkarenwinkfield.com/radio-talk Accessed 11 December 2015

[18] ICT University www.mbarika.com Accessed 7 January 2016

[19] Ferlay J, Steliarova-Foucher E, Lortet-Tieulent J, Rosso S, Coebergh J W, Comber H, Forman D and Bray F 2013 Cancer incidence and mortality patterns in Europe: estimates for 40 countries in 2012 *Eur. J. Cancer* **49** 1374–1403

[20] Williams M J, Otero I V and Harford J B 2013 Evaluation of the impact of NCI's Summer Curriculum on Cancer Prevention on participants from low- and middle-income countries *J. Cancer Educ.* **28** 27–32

[21] Ngwa W 2015 Potential for information and communication technologies to catalyze global collaborations in radiation oncology *Int. J. Radiat. Oncol. Biol. Phys.* **91** 444–7

[22] Elzawawy A 2012 Science and affordability of cancer drugs and radiotherapy in the world—win–win scenarios *Advances in Cancer Management* ed; Ravinder Mohan (Rijeka: InTech)

[23] Diaspora for development in Africa http://siteresources.worldbank.org/EXTDECPROSPECTS/Resources/476882-1157133580628/DfD_FullReport.pdf Accessed 7 January 2016

[24] In Sudan, efforts to erase breast cancer stigma www.futurity.org/in-sudan-efforts-to-erase-breast-cancer-stigma Accessed 3 January 2016

[25] Mohammed S I, Williams C K, Ndom P and Holland J F 2012 The African Organization for Research and Training in Cancer: historical perspective, *Curr. Oncol.* **19** 272–6

[26] Adewole I 2014 Building capacity for sustainable research programmes for cancer in Africa *Nat. Rev. Clinical Oncol.* **11** 251–9

[27] Cavalli F and Atun R 2015 Towards a global cancer fund *Lancet Oncol.* **16** 133–4

[28] Report on regional workshop to raise awareness on medical physicists' roles in ensuring safety in imaging- with emphasis on pediatric imaging (Dar es Salaam, Republic of Tanzania, 26–28 November 2014) www.wfpiweb.org/Portals/7/Child%20Imaging%20Safety/Dar_WHO_Regional_workshop_report.pdf

[29] Walt B 2010 As technology surges, radiation safeguards lag www.nytimes.com/2010/01/27/us/27radiation.html?hpw Accessed 3 January 2016

IOP Publishing

Wilfred Ngwa and Twalib Ngoma

Chapter 5

Low cost technologies for global radiation oncology

Kind words do not cost much. Yet they accomplish much.
Blaise Pascal [1]

5.1 State-of-the-art lower cost technologies in radiation oncology

Radiotherapy is often considered to be an expensive treatment modality. One of the adverse perceptions or misleading assumptions is that its deployment in LMIC is not feasible. Studies [2, 3] have indicated that radiotherapy is a relatively cost-effective treatment intervention. Although substantial investment and a number of skilled professionals are needed initially, a positive return on this is expected in the longer term. In addition, radiotherapy is crucial for the effective treatment of over half of cancer patients. Without it, these patients will die and suffer unnecessarily. In LMIC, after factoring in all the levels of cost related to the procurement, maintenance and operation of a machine, minus the costs for physicians, estimates place the median cost per fraction at 4.87 US dollars for a cobalt machine and 11.02 US dollars for a LINAC.

However, when the price of radiotherapy treatment is compared to LMIC incomes, it can be unaffordable for many patients, especially since most of them have no health insurance. This is what unfortunately foments the adverse perception that radiotherapy is not feasible for LMIC. It is therefore necessary to continue to find ways to significantly lower the cost of radiotherapy, including via the development of technologies that can lower: (a) the upfront costs of developing a new facility, including those for building, equipment and the training of new staff, and (b) the operating costs for delivering treatment once the facility has been established.

doi:10.1088/978-0-7503-1224-0ch5

Cognizant of this need, and the growing global cancer burden, which disproportionately affects LMIC, the IAEA's PACT established the Advisory Group on Increasing Access to Radiotherapy Technology in LMIC (AGaRT) [2]. The purpose of this program is to engage manufacturers, users and experts in finding the way forward to expand radiotherapy facilities: discovering affordable, suitable and sustainable solutions to address the shortfall of radiotherapy machines in LMIC, with costs being a major factor. At the 2015 Harvard summit, the PACT director highlighted some of the key factors to take into consideration for sustainable solutions:

- appropriate, affordable and suitable equipment compliant with the international safety and quality standards;
- innovative and cost-effective radiotherapy solutions, including optimization of financial schemes for radiotherapy, suitable for use in LMIC;
- relevant workforce requirements for operating radiotherapy equipment;
- awareness of the role of radiotherapy technology in cancer treatment and palliation, including global advocacy efforts in line with other global initiatives;
- development of economic assessment tools;
- adoption of AGaRT-recommended basic radiotherapy equipment package in LMIC.

More affordable radiotherapy equipment with guaranteed functionality for many years includes: (a) megavoltage treatment units; (b) simulators (x-ray or CT); (c) brachytherapy treatment units; (d) dosimetry equipment for QA shielding blocks and port films; and (e) immobilization devices. Some manufacturers have released newer technologies that are relatively affordable, and efforts are being made to do more in this direction, as this is urgently needed given the growing cancer burden and the tragic disparities in radiation oncology services. Here are some examples.

TeamBest

TeamBest [4], which started as Best Medical International, was founded in 1977 in Springfield, Virginia, USA by Indo-American engineer Krishnan Suthanthiran. Initially, the company offered one high-quality product, the Iridium-192 brachytherapy seed strand. Today, TeamBest offers many radiotherapy products and services, which are represented in North America, Europe, Latin America, Africa, the Middle East and Asia. TeamBest's stated goal is to reduce healthcare costs by controlling the supply chain and manufacturing costs.

One of TeamBest's best-known lower-cost technologies/solutions is the Best® Gamma Teletherapy™ system, or Theratron, which uses cobalt-60, with significantly lower initial investment and operating costs relative to LINACs. The Theratron specifications indicate that it can be operated using generator or solar power, that it can operate on 115 V AC or 230 V AC single phase and that it requires no special cooling. Recent updates indicate that Theratrons can now be equipped or upgraded with the latest intensity modulated radiotherapy (IMRT), image guided radiotherapy (IGRT) and stereotactic

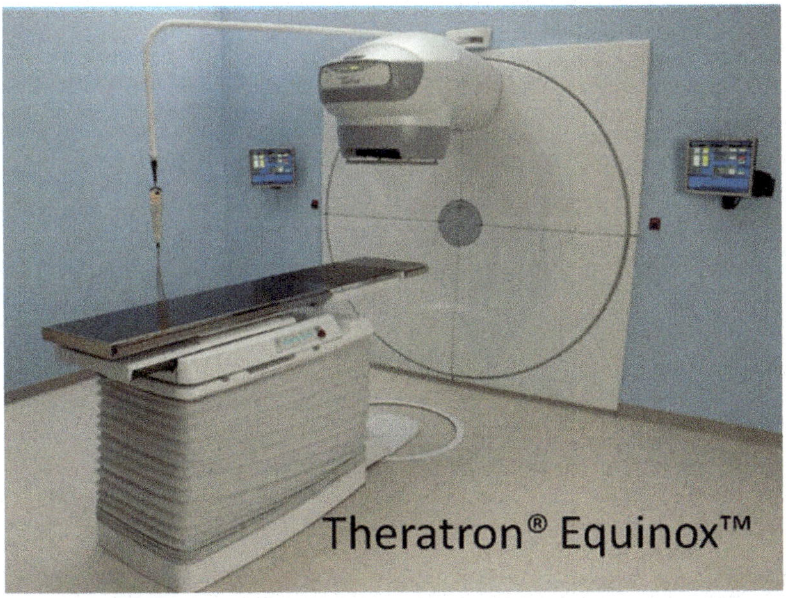

Figure 5.1. The Theratron Equinox. Reproduced with permission from TeamBest.

radiosurgery (SRS) technologies, e.g. a multi-leaf collimator (MLC) for IMRT and kV- or MV-based IGRT solutions. TeamBest presents their cobalt machines as being simpler to use, with reduced maintenance, running costs and downtime.

The Theratron is best for head, neck, breast and skin cancer, as well as palliative care. In addition, with the MLCs now available, advanced IMRT cancer treatments can be performed with these cobalt units. The Theratron® Equinox™ (figure 5.1) is presented as the most advanced isotope-based teletherapy system available on the market. The machine is designed to facilitate advanced treatment techniques and reduces treatment times with many time-saving features.

The cobalt systems offer a reduced quality assurance burden and reduced staff demands, while they also require less auxiliary infrastructure to run (e.g. power supply in a city or remote area) and less maintenance, which is usually a very desirable future in LMIC.

Given the potential for using ICTs in e.g. telemedicine, as described in the previous chapter, it is also worth noting that cobalt teletherapy units require less support from medical physicists for calibration, and therefore ICTs could be used more readily by medical physicists to provide information and guidance remotely when needed. In LMIC where there are often less than a handful of medical physicists for the whole country, remote support may be very helpful including remote training.

Best Theratronics' products are available in over 100 countries, with over 2700 teletherapy units worldwide. More information and a comprehensive listing of other company products can be found on the company website[1].

[1] www.teambest.com/products.html.

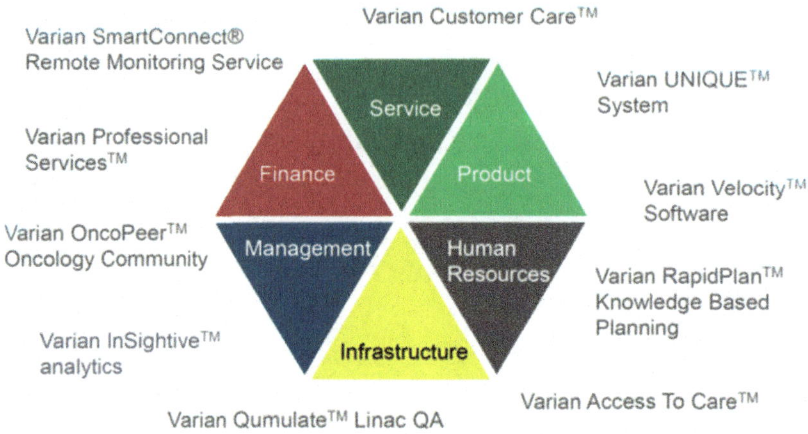

Figure 5.2. Varian Medical technologies.

Varian Medical Systems

Varian Medical Systems [5] was founded in 1948 by Russell H Varian, Sigurd F Varian, William Webster Hansen and Edward Ginzton to sell the Klystron (the first tube that could amplify and leverage electromagnetic waves at microwave frequencies) and other electromagnetic equipment. It has now grown into a leading radiation oncology technology company for LINACs and associated software. In line with the IAEA AGaRT initiative, manufacturers like Varian Medical Systems have released new LINACs (4–6 MeV) that include the basic capabilities and software to provide an integrated treatment system [2]. It has been noted that these systems also include a warranty and training to educate operators in system use [2]. One noteworthy solution introduced by Varian Medical Systems is the UNIQUE™, which they present as the world's first low-energy radiotherapy system with image-guidance and RapidArc treatment capabilities [2], making advanced care more affordable and more widely available to cancer patients around the world. Varian describes this system as 'a comprehensive, cost-effective offering that provides cancer patients with standard treatments as well as advanced techniques, including IMRT, IGRT, and RapidArc® treatments'. Varian also offers a version of this solution without the RapidArc technology or image-guidance software, for centers that prefer to begin with a more basic yet upgradeable platform that is cheaper.

Since its launch, the UNIQUE™ low-energy platform has been rolled out globally, with installations in many European, Asian, Latin American and African countries.

Varian Medical Systems also have a number of platform technologies that could be employed to facilitate global radiation oncology. For example, Qumulate™ (figure 5.2) is a LINAC tool that allows clinics to visualize, store and manage their quality assurance machine data using a modern, cloud-based application. Through an easily accessible web application, clinics can create quality assurance templates and monitor their machine performance metrics, comparing them with those of other machines. The Varian Velocity^{TM} software can also enable remote treatment planning. More information on Varian Medical Systems and products can be found on their website[2].

Elekta

Elekta [6] was founded in 1972 by Lars Leksell in Sweden to commercialize the development of the Leksell Stereotactic System and the Leksell Gamma Knife, which he had researched and developed. Since then, Elekta has expanded into a leading human care company pioneering significant innovations and clinical solutions for treating cancer and brain disorders. The company now develops sophisticated, state-of-the-art tools and treatment-planning systems for radiation therapy, radiosurgery and brachytherapy.

The Elekta Compact^{TM} [7] has been profiled as one of the cost-effective solutions released by Elekta in recent years. It constitutes a flexible yet affordable compact LINAC, with a small footprint and a cost-effective design, which could be attractive 'for oncology centers that need to start small, but are thinking big for the future'. It has been designed to be a dependable, high throughput system for busy treatment centers. The operation of this system is relatively simple and it is reliable, allowing more patients to be treated quickly and effectively. With its modular design, upgrades and new functions and features can be added easily, making it a robust standalone solution for radiation therapy.

With respect to ICT or telemedicine, one of Elekta's products, the Elekta IntelliMax™, can be employed to facilitate remote support capabilities to ensure optimized equipment availability and fine-tuned clinical performance. In addition, as institutions become more collaborative and treatments become more personalized, Elekta has developed cutting-edge software, MOSAIQ, which enables remote access to complete clinical and patient information, with better tools for sharing, analyzing and applying information, making it easier to tap into the knowledge and experience of remote collaborators. More information on Elekta and products can be found at the website[3].

The Bhabhatron

The Bhabhatron [8] is a signature radiotherapy technology that was developed in India to serve as an affordable solution for radiation therapy in that LMIC. The technology was developed by the Bhabha Atomic Research Centre (BARC) as a sophisticated telecobalt machine. It is the outcome of a collaboration between BARC and Panacea Medical Technologies Pvt Ltd, India. It has been profiled as not only being less expensive, but also incorporating a number of safety and automation features, with the potential to make safe and affordable radiation therapy accessible to the citizens of India and many other countries. An advanced version of the Bhabhatron (BH-II) incorporates MLCs, allowing it to be used for 3D conformal

[2] www.varian.com.

[3] www.elekta.com.

treatments. The BH II is also equipped with enhanced features such as a motorized wedge, auto-setup, asymmetric collimation, a computer console, an advanced radiolucent patient couch, an electromechanical and software-based anti-collision device, an auto-closure mechanism during emergencies and a remote diagnostic facility for assisting a proactive maintenance schedule. The remote diagnostic facility could also be very valuable for centers with limited human capacity. More information on the Bhabhatron can be found at the website[4].

The above examples are only a sample of profiles for lower-cost radiotherapy machines.

LINAC versus cobalt

One of the questions often asked when planning to establish a radiotherapy service today, especially in LMIC, is whether to purchase a LINAC or a cobalt unit. Massoud Samiei, a former director of the IAEA PACT program recently published an excellent discussion of this question [2]. His article reported that cobalt-60 units have customarily been considered to be the more robust workhorses to place in new cancer clinics in LMIC, because of the lower upfront cost and the fact that they are easier to operate for treatment delivery, planning and maintenance. He noted, however, that cobalt machines have become more sophisticated and that their prices have increased as they incorporate other advanced features, such as MLCs. There are also security concerns, especially since the 11 September 2001 attack in the USA, which have made the transport and return of spent cobalt-60 sources more complicated. For cobalt machines, which have a useful life of ~20 years, the main issue today is the need to replace the cobalt-60 source every five to six years, which could cost ~150 000 US dollars [2]. Regular disposal of the old sources also costs money, ~250 000 to ~350 000 US dollars, unless prior arrangements are made during procurement. Special authorization and licensing is required for cobalt-60 sources from other countries in transit, unless the supplier is able to use international routes and direct transport means [2].

Meanwhile, for LINACs, a few manufactures, including those described above, are now putting lower-cost LINACs onto the market, which could benefit LMIC. LINACs can typically be operated for over ten years before replacement, but the capital or upfront costs are still relatively high. These become even higher when other costs are taken into account, e.g. commissioning, operation, training, QA programs, maintenance, and so forth.

Therefore, the choice between cobalt and LINAC is increasingly dependent on the buyer or LMIC's radiotherapy experience, the financial and technical capacity, and the available workforce. According to Samiei, for most LMIC, having operated and used cobalt machines for a number of years, a mixed choice of both cobalt-60 and LINAC machines is probably the right approach, where resources are available.

[4] www.barc.gov.in/clip/bhabhatron.html

Other lower cost radiotherapy tech

In addition to radiotherapy machines, other companies present themselves as providing affordable and effective technologies that can be employed in developing countries for radiation oncology. For example, PTW Freiburg GmbH [9] in Germany offers dosimetry and quality assurance solutions for radiotherapy. These include patient plan verification solutions, e.g. in the Octavius series of modular solutions for 4D and 2D IMRT quality assurance. There are also other radiotherapy technologies that could facilitate the treatment of patients in many LMIC.

5.2 Emerging lower-cost technologies in radiation oncology

The stark reality is that, even with the available lower-cost radiotherapy infrastructure, and with no downtime, power outages or maintenance issues, the costs for radiotherapy are still not affordable for most LMIC populations. Affordability is inseparably linked to value, quality, efficiency, equity and accessibility. One must therefore also address healthcare systems overall when dealing with this. With the growing global radiation oncology movement, it is now important for physicists, engineers and other radiation oncology health professionals to work together to develop more affordable solutions. This could also involve partnerships with industry to develop new low-cost technologies that can facilitate affordability and access. The National Cancer Institute has a number of funding mechanisms to promote the development of low-cost technologies, although the funding opportunities are still limited. The overall goal of this funding is to increase the availability of low-cost portable technologies for cancer diagnosis, imaging and treatment in LMIC. Partnerships and collaborations will be very important in this effort to develop lower-cost technologies and more affordable adaptations. Industry–academic/research institution partnerships could be an important driver of this. The United States National Cancer Institute center for global health particularly encourages ‘twinning’ partnerships between comprehensive cancer centers in the United States and partners in LMIC. The annual GHC summit at Harvard is now actively promoting or facilitating such partnerships and working to highlight emerging lower-cost technologies for global radiation oncology, as well as the use of ICTs to facilitate access and affordability, as highlighted in the previous chapter.

Table 5.1 highlights some lower-cost technologies that are emerging or being developed for radiation oncology. One example is a ‘Low-cost enabling technology for image-guided photodynamic therapy of oral cancer’ by Hempstead *et al* [10]. This project was funded through the Nation Cancer Institute grant mechanism for low-cost technologies, with physicist Dr Jonathan Celli of the Massachusetts General Hospital and University of Massachusetts Boston being the principal investigator (PI). In their work, the PI and his collaborators are developing a low-cost enabling technology to extend the clinical benefit of photodynamic therapy (PDT) to regions with little or no access to electricity or medical infrastructure. They have demonstrated the efficacy of a device based on a 635 nm wavelength high-output LED powered by three AA disposable alkaline batteries to achieve a strong cytotoxic response in monolayer and 3D cultures of A431 squamous carcinoma cells following photosensitization through

Table 5.1. Examples of emerging low-cost technologies for global radiation oncology.

Emerging technology	Potential application/reference
HEC detector	A new low-cost x-ray radiation detector [14].
Low-cost enabling technology for image-guided photodynamic therapy of oral cancer	Low-cost photodynamic therapy devices for global health settings: characterization of battery-powered LED performance and smartphone imaging in 3D tumor models [10].
TiDTaC	Devices designed to halve or substantially reduce radiotherapy treatment/waiting times with minimal collateral damage to healthy tissue (Ngwa *et al* www.tidtac.org)
NanoX	A compact radiotherapy system intended to lower the costs of building and operating a radiotherapy center (Keall *et al* http://medicalphysicsweb.org/cws/article/research/51692)
High-Z nanoparticles	Targeted radiotherapy with high-Z nanoparticles [12]
Glass beads	Low-cost commercial glass beads used as dosimeters in radiotherapy [15]
RO-ILS	An online portal that allows radiation oncology centers to provide non-patient-specific data about the radiation therapy near-misses and safety incidents that have occurred at their facility in a secure, non-punitive environment (ASTRO/AAPM)
SpekCalc	x-ray spectra calculation program; it quickly and accurately calculates photon x-ray spectra in the range 0–300 kV for a variety of filtration materials
CERR	A software platform for developing and sharing research results in radiation therapy treatment planning
Brainlab's Quentry	An online platform for image transfer, sharing and collaboration. Built on a secure, HIPAA-compliant infrastructure, Quentry supports clinicians throughout the referral, diagnosis, planning and treatment workflow. Physicians can join and connect with each other for free and build a medical referral network, for either individual or hospital use

administration of aminolevulinic acid (ALA) to induce the accumulation of protoporphyrin IX (PpIX). Further motivated by the well-established capacity of PDT photosensitizers to serve as tumor-selective fluorescence contrast agents, these scientists demonstrated the ability of a consumer smartphone with low-cost add-ons to measure concentration-dependent PpIX fluorescence, laying the groundwork for the ongoing development of image-guided ALA-PDT treatment technologies for global health applications.

While the Celli group's work is at much higher wavelengths than x-rays, it may be possible to leverage the similar high-wavelength photons that were recently discovered to be present during radiotherapy in the form of Cerenkov radiation to substantially boost the damage to cancer cells while minimizing healthy tissue toxicity. This technology is under development by the tiny drones to target cancer (TiDTaC) group led by Wilfred Ngwa at Harvard Medical School and the University of Massachusetts [11]. TiDTaCs are designed to substantially reduce radiotherapy treatment times, while at the same time minimizing any collateral damage to cancer patients. Such technology could be particularly beneficial for patients in LMIC countries, where waiting times can be long due to the lack of radiotherapy infrastructure increase [2]. The dearth or lack of radiotherapy units in many LMIC causes prolonged waiting times to receive treatment and can even affect the timing between the administration of radiotherapy doses, which can seriously compromise clinical outcomes and treatment effectiveness. The smart TiDTaC technology is profiled as a rice-size device that incorporates a potent combination of microscopic nanoparticles and/or immunoadjuvants, which can be released locally to amplify damage to cancer cells. This could provide the equivalent effect of stereotactic ablative radiotherapy (SABR) through these programmed nanoparticles. Hence, instead of treating patients with many fractions, these low-cost devices could replace currently used radiotherapy biomaterials (fiducials and spacers) for highly localized radiation boosting with minimal toxicity to healthy tissues. The TiDTaCs represent an advanced but lower-cost version of radiotherapy application with *in situ* dose-painting (RAiD), as described by the same scientists previously [12]. Ongoing research could make TiDTaCs an alternative to making cobalt machines more like LINACs, or LINACs more like cobalt machines.

Another example of a technology worth highlighting comes from Zygmanski *et al* [13] who developed prototypes for a new low-cost high-energy current (HEC) x-ray radiation detector. Based on the experimental results for a 100 ms sampling time, the scientists showed that it is possible to measure the time dependence of x-ray beams for an x-ray tube current of 0.1 mA or higher. The HEC device has significant advantages: the generation of its signal does not require an external power supply; it can be made in any size and shape, including flexible curvilinear forms; and it is inexpensive. It remains to be determined which potential applications in medical dosimetry (both *in vivo* and external) or radiation protection would benefit from such self-powered detectors. Once development has been completed, this could be a very useful technology in LMIC.

Another technology that can be further adapted for LMIC is the Radiation Oncology Incident Learning System™ (RO-ILS), which was developed by ASTRO and AAPM as an online portal that will allow radiation oncology centers to provide non-patient-specific data about the radiation therapy near-misses and safety incidents that have occurred at their facility in a secure, non-punitive environment. According to ASTRO, data collected in RO-ILS can be used to educate the radiation oncology community about how to improve safety and patient care. An adaptation of this that is applicable to LMIC would be very useful, because as more radiation technologies become available in LMIC, a silent crisis of safety is developing. No fee is charged for radiation therapy centers to use the RO-ILS platform, and it can be used as a standalone incident learning system or to complement an institution's existing system.

In general, lower-cost technologies have the potential to change the lives of millions of individuals living in LMIC. With the emerging global radiation oncology movement, physicists, engineers and other scientists must also now focus on developing such technologies, or adaptations of current technologies, that can make radiotherapy more affordable and accessible in LMIC. The development of such technologies could lead to what are called trickle-up innovations, where such technologies developed with an LMIC focus find their way into the developed world. An example of this from another field is GE Healthcare's Ultrasound Vscan technology, originally designed for LMIC and later commercialized as a low-cost alternative for emergency medical technicians and emergency rooms in industrialized countries. Such trickle-up innovations occur when a designer can focus on and adapt the design parameters for LMIC.

In the effort to develop lower-cost technology, collaborations with LMIC partners are strongly encouraged, with appropriate feedback to optimize the application. The development of these technologies should also be based on co-creation, with specific end-user adoptability and feedback. These should be incorporated to optimize designs so that effectiveness and durability in the intended clinical setting are ensured. Collaborations and co-creation with LMIC end-users can be powerful in allowing collaborators from various disciplines, institutions and sectors to innovate around the challenges currently faced in global radiation oncology. These in turn can act as an impetus towards developing specific solutions for the intended user to successfully translate their research.

References

[1] www.brainyquote.com/quotes/quotes/b/blaisepasc159858.html Accessed 3 January 2016

[2] Samiei M 2013 Challenges of making radiotherapy accessible in developing countries *Cancer Control* **2013** 85–94

[3] Atun R 2015 Expanding global access to radiotherapy *Lancet Oncol.* **16** 1153–86

[4] *TeamBest* www.teambest.com/about.html

[5] *Varian Medical* https://en.wikipedia.org/wiki/Varian_Medical_Systems

[6] *Elekta* https://en.wikipedia.org/wiki/Elekta

[7] *Elekta Compact* www.elekta.com/radiotherapy/treatment-delivery-systems/elekta-compact.html Accessed 17 December 2016

[8] *Bhabhatron* www.panaceamedical.com/bhabhatron.php

[9] *PTW* www.ptw.de

[10] Hempstead J, Jones D P, Ziouche A, Cramer G M, Rizvi I, Arnason S, Hasan T and Celli J P 2015 Low-cost photodynamic therapy devices for global health settings: characterization of battery-powered LED performance and smartphone imaging in 3D tumor models *Sci. Rep* **5** 10093

[11] *TiDTaC* www.tidtac.org

[12] Ngwa W, Kumar R, Sridhar S, Korideck H, Zygmanski P, Cormack R A, Berbeco R and Makrigiorgos G M 2014 Targeted radiotherapy with gold nanoparticles: current status and future perspectives *Nanomedicine* **9** 1063–82

[13] Zygmanski P, Shrestha S, Briovio D, Karellas A and Sajo E 2016 Prototypes of self-powered radiation detectors employing intrinsic high-energy current *Med. Phys.* **43** 16

[14] Zygmanski P, Shrestha S, Elshahat B, Karellas A and Sajo E 2015 Dosimetric properties of high energy current (HEC) detector in keV x-ray beams *Phys. Med. Biol.* **60** N121–9

[15] Jafari S M, Bradley D A, Gouldstone C A, Sharpe P H G, Alalawi A, Jordan T J, Clark C H, Nisbet A and Spyrou N M 2014 Low-cost commercial glass beads as dosimeters in radiotherapy *Radiat. Phys. Chem.* **97** 95–101

IOP Publishing

Emerging Models for Global Health in Radiation Oncology

Wilfred Ngwa and Twalib Ngoma

Chapter 6

Global radiation oncology made simpler: a practical guide and recommendations for high-impact radiation oncology global health

In the moment of crisis, the wise build bridges and the foolish build dams.
Nigerian proverb

6.1 Making it easier to participate in global radiation oncology

With growing interest in global health, one key issue is how to make it easier for people to participate in global health collaborations. Some of the ways to overcome the barriers to global health were highlighted in previous chapters, including the use of ICTs to overcome space–time barriers. However, according to many global health leaders, there is much more that can be done.

Lowering the activation energy for participation
To catalyze participation, it is necessary to make it easier to become involved or get started. In order to get started, people need to know what is going on, and where. The National Cancer Institute Center for Global Health recently partnered with Global Oncology, Inc. to develop a web-based tool designed to facilitate cancer research and control activity planning. This tool, called the Global Cancer Project Map (GCPM), is a database that allows users to locate and learn more about international cancer projects and research programs through the use of an interactive world map. The GCPM employs detailed search functionalities to streamline searches for cancer research and control programs, training activities and capacity-building initiatives. It is available to users free of charge and is accessible from anywhere in the world online[1].

[1] http://globalonc.org/Projects/global-cancer-project-map.

doi:10.1088/978-0-7503-1224-0ch6

Table 6.1. Examples of funding mechanisms that can support career development pathways in global radiation oncology.

Funding source	Description
NIH career development (K-level) awards	www.grants.nih.gov/training/careerdevelopmentawards.htm
Fogarty International Research Scientist Development Award	www.fic.nih.gov/Programs/Pages/research-scientists.aspx
Yamagiwa-Yoshida Memorial international study grants	www.uicc.org/programmes/geti/our-activities/study-grants
ASCO Conquer Cancer Foundation Young Investigator Award	www.conquercancerfoundation.org/young-investigator-award
ASTRO Junior Faculty Career Research Training Award	www.astro.org/Research/Funding-Opportunities/ASTRO-Supported-Grants/Junior-Faculty/Index.aspx
Varian Medical Systems research grant	www.varian.com/us/corporate/research_programs/research_grants.html
Elekta research grants	www.elekta.com/company/programs/elekta-research-grants.html
Grants.gov	A site where the US government pools all grants opportunities in one place

In addition to the GCPM, the National Cancer Institute Center for Global Health and other funding agencies, such as Fogarty international, have a listing of funding mechanisms, including non-NIH funding opportunities [1], that could help seed collaborations once people find appropriate partners, e.g. from the GCPM. One such opportunity from Fogarty is a new LMIC junior faculty award (table 6.1). This career development award for LMIC scientists provides support to enable recipients to conduct mentored research and career development activities. The awards will require input from mentors in both a developed and a developing country, who are both accomplished investigators in the proposed research area and experienced in guiding independent investigators. Fogarty also runs an International Research Scientist Development Award, which targets US scientists interested in global health (table 6.1).

Another way to facilitate participation in global radiation oncology is via knowledge sharing. The Consortium of Universities for Global Health (CUGH) [2] has as part of its mission statement the aim to facilitate the sharing of knowledge to address global health challenges. CUGH assists its members in sharing their expertise across education, research and service and is dedicated to creating equity and reducing health disparities everywhere. CUGH conferences are an attractive yearly feature for global health. Increasingly, AAPM and ASTRO are also organizing knowledge-sharing symposia at their annual conferences, which can also facilitate networking and the building of partnerships.

Note that there are many other funding sources for global health, e.g. grants.gov, that those interested in global health can take advantage of, including typical career development grants, which may provide protected time from clinical or other duties to conduct research and secure global health experience in other countries.

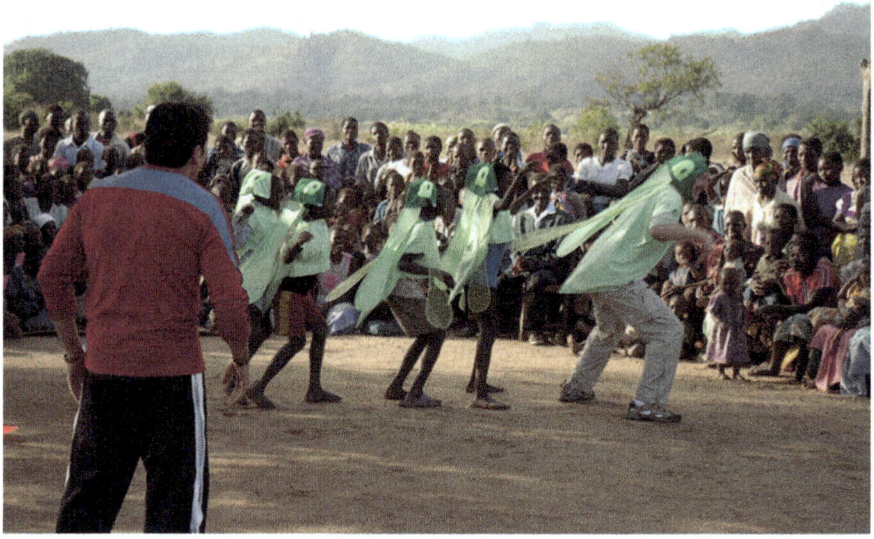

Figure 6.1. Blending in with Malawian culture.

6.2 Facilitating high-impact outcomes

After collaborations are initiated, it is important to make sure they are successful and can be appropriately sustained. Some issues that need to be addressed to ensure sustainability and/or high impact include fundamental ones, such as authorship, patents, ethics, culture, etc. It is important to prepare those who are engaging in global health to be able to deal with such issues. Even when the goal is to cure cancer or save lives, such fundamental issues, if not addressed, can lead to a poor experience or low-impact collaborations.

Culture and respect

The experience of an influential and wealthy American who had a dream, and an ambitious plan, to channel vast humanitarian aid from the USA to communities in Africa illustrates some of these issues. The *Wall Street Journal* [3] published a lengthy article on how the African dream of this man and his good intentions turned into a nightmare. This dream was to dramatically improve the lot of one million orphans in Africa. The plan was to house orphans in a facility that was to be an orphanage, bed-and-breakfast, game reserve, college, industrial park and Disneyesque tourist destination. From the analysis of many who followed this story, there were a number of compounding factors or mistakes that made the project fail [4]. Those who are planning to engage in or are engaged in global health may learn something from these mistakes.

1. The inevitable clash of cultures. The orphanages (dream villages) that the American wanted to establish were at variance with the African culture of kinship and caring for their members, and there was a need to engage better

with the local population to find a mutually acceptable pathway. The American did not even listen to the local US ambassador, who lauded the initiative to help the orphans but advised that his countryman execute the project in a way that did not conflict with the local culture by moving the orphans away from their own villages to the dream village he was creating. So there is a need to respect local cultures in any collaboration, no matter the good intentions, even if it is a project to cure cancer.

2. Excessive demands or expectations. The American demanded major tracts of land, while land is arguably one of the most prized possessions of and a national asset for Africans. Demands or expectations like these can be unrealistic, especially if the project does not give equal or appropriate credit to the locals. The land issue can be a particularly sensitive issue for some LMIC, who were colonized. Referring to the American, one op-ed writer in the local newspaper wrote, 'Why can't he simply tell us that he wants to be given the whole country so that he can gloat to his friends overseas that he owns a modern day colony in Africa…?' [5]. This highlights an issue where the non-LMIC partner is just interested in receiving credit for the work they are doing, especially if they are bringing the funding.

This is just one of many stories in which people with good intentions, e.g. for global health, may be hampered because of a fundamental lack of understanding of other cultures, or because they are driven by their own agendas and the credit they expect to receive. From the details of the story, the following recommendations can be made.

1. Do not arrive in LMIC to execute your noble project with a know-it-all mentality.
2. Respect the local culture and even blend in.
3. Treat the LMIC participants as equal partners and also acknowledge them equally in any outcomes to share credit.

In a *Science* article, 'Balancing the collaboration equation' [6], Jon Cohen emphasized the importance of equality, and not the customary and inherent inequalities that can cause tensions in collaborations, including situations where locals may not even be included in research publications for which they contributed data. Cohen noted that LMIC researchers often find themselves balancing their expectations and needs with those of their developed country peers, who often provide the bulk of the funding, but also have better access to organizers of conferences, journal editors and the international media. The collaboration must be viewed as a give-and-take, mutually beneficial partnership. Friedman *et al*, a working group of the Association of Schools of Public Health Global Health Committee, emphasized in a *Lancet* article that global health should not always be perceived as international aid, with technologies and interventions flowing from the wealthier developed countries of the Global North to the poorer countries of the Global South [7]. *Science* [6] visited a dozen projects in LMIC and noted that the tensions which characterized collaborative efforts, mostly revolved around equity: access to financial resources and facilities, participation, transfer of technology, self-reliance, training opportunities, and credit. Developed country partners also occasionally confront their LMIC colleagues about using lab resources to conduct personal business.

Diaspora involvement

Another recommendation for facilitating high-impact collaborations is to involve the diaspora. Outreach involvement of the diaspora would, arguably, spawn and catalyze greater impact collaborations and help turn the brain drain into a gain against cancer. The diaspora's passion for contributing to their original countries, their better appreciation of both Western and sending country cultures, and their substantial human resource and financial potential (e.g. over 50 billion US dollars per year in remittances made by the African Diaspora) could be a significant asset, including for supporting crowdfunding. In 2014, remittances to sub-Saharan Africa amounted to 67.1 billion US dollars according to the African Economic Outlook [8].

Professional development pathway

Another recommendation discussed is the proposal for a new academic or professional development pathway for global radiation oncology [9] made by Olson *et al.* The authors highlight the fact that while radiation oncology trainees are showing increased interest in global health, the transition from being a trainee interested in global oncology to becoming junior faculty is not well established. At the 2015 GHC summit, global health leaders also encouraged radiation oncology department chairs to create professional development pathways for staff or faculty looking to incorporate global health as a major career activity. Some of these pathways can be supported by the funding highlighted in table 6.1. Olson *et al* noted that radiation oncology health professionals starting a career in global health need protected time or a start-up period consistent with that of traditional clinical and basic researchers. This will allow people to focus on the project, with better outcomes anticipated. The ICEC [10] has proposed that academic advancement take the following criteria into account in global health: scholarship, education, policy and infrastructure development, metrics and mentorship. In the years ahead, these criteria or adaptations thereof will be helpful to facilitate the growing field of global radiation oncology

Research administration

It is also highly recommended that LMIC institutions create research administrative infrastructure to facilitate collaborations and address key areas in grant management, such as fiscal accountability, data management, research oversight and the submission of grant applications. These should be established, particularly at the hubs of excellence, with local institutional ownership and commitment to sustain and integrate these activities into their overall strategic plan for research support. Furthermore, the hubs of excellence are encouraged to work at and strengthen the capacity for research administration at other regional institutes that lack this component. Research administration is particularly recommended for funded consortia.

Crowdsourcing

It is also important to provide opportunities for sharing ideas, to continue to improve global health programs or collaborations. Such engagement can provide a crucible for new ideas and continued progress, encourage input from the younger generation and help provide more perspective to enhance global radiation oncology. One example is that of the Global Health Delivery program at Harvard [11], which regularly gets those in the field or frontline to provide input on different topics. This input is disseminated through multiple channels, including open-access online professional communities, case studies, educational programs and scholarly publications, with the overall mission to build a network of professionals dedicated to improving the delivery of value-based health care globally. The platform is open to input and participation from anyone who is interested.

Crowdsourcing is one of the avenues where the diaspora can also complement efforts in global oncology. The diaspora can help to provide input and support work to address the primary level disparities in cancer education and prevention, as well as the stigma associated with cancer in Africa. The diaspora can also be crowdsourced for the development of appropriate words for cancer where there is a vocabulary deficit and the translation of content from developed countries into appropriate language with a suitable cultural context to better communicate information in their native LMIC.

Publications/dissemination

It is recommended that the funders of global radiation oncology research require that all work supported by them be open access, so that LMIC researchers can also access and appear in public digital libraries, preferably at the time of publication and without constraints of copyright. Universities and other research institutions should foster compliance with such policies from funding agencies and supplement those policies with institution-based repositories of publications and databases. Issues of authorship should also be addressed right at the beginning of the partnerships.

Research institutions should also develop novel approaches, e.g. simplified web-based procedures for executing agreements like materials transfer and nondisclosure agreements, in order to expedite the sharing of information and research materials with partners in LMIC.

Platforms like the Global Health Catalyst should aggregate the published literature, incorporate unpublished databases or clinical trial information, promote digital collaboration and disseminate news and other information about common interests in radiation oncology.

While generating new knowledge, the existing knowledge on global radiation should be regularly shared. Besides the regular global health summits at Harvard, the AAPM and ASTRO could encourage greater global health activity at annual conferences and create an abstract submission category for global health. Greater dissemination of knowledge on the benefits of global health oncology and impact awareness would also be greatly beneficial in moving the field forward and attracting greater investment. Global health research involves not only generating knowledge relevant to the context of LMIC, but also effectively transferring such knowledge and technologies to LMIC settings and ensuring that it is applied on a sustained basis. With research increasingly conducted globally through virtual communities of geographically dispersed scientists, it is critically important that any information exchange promotes sustainable international research partnerships and enables the timely dissemination of best practices.

Patenting and intellectual property

It is recommended that research institutions consider adopting patent policies and licensing practices that enable and encourage the development of technologies to create products for which traditional market forces are not sufficient. Patent policies should also ensure that LMIC partners are recognized, even if they do not provide funding. Some of these patentable intellectual properties should be particularly encouraged in joint research projects, e.g. in the development of lower-cost technologies.

Brain drain

It is recommended that governments and other entities work together more to understand and improve the dynamics of the labor market to stem the tide of workforce migration. Such work may require commitments by governments to construct and finance sound human resource plans, with potential support via external donor assistance and cooperation. The poor working conditions that can drive the brain drain or create disincentives for health workers to perform at the highest level should be addressed.

Advocacy

Advocacy efforts are especially recommended for better patient safety. Recent workshops and surveys [12] have highlighted major patient safety issues in the use of radiation technologies in LMIC. When the *New York Times* reported on such incidences in the USA [13], there was a major outcry, leading to testimony in the US Congress by AAPM and ASTRO representatives to address the issue. Imagine the situation where many African countries do not even have a medical physicist, coupled with a dramatic increase in the use of radiation technologies, including for diagnostic imaging. It is crucial to raise public awareness, as the *New York Times* did, and advocate for the recognition of the importance of medical physicists in ensuring the safety of patients, healthcare staff and the general public when using such technologies. The benefits of this will go beyond cancer treatment, as radiation technologies are widely used in diagnostic testing for other diseases, including cardiovascular disease, infectious disease, trauma, musculoskeletal disorders, dentistry, etc. In fact, the absence or shortage of medical physicists in African countries is a silent healthcare crisis, which is likely affecting even policy makers and their family members, even if they are unaware of it. Greater advocacy in this area could shed light on this and bolster efforts to train more medical physicists and radiation medicine staff, who are badly needed in these countries. This could in turn benefit global radiation oncology. If there was an outcry in the United States, where there is already a relatively high level of patient safety, then an even bigger outcry is needed in LMIC to inform policy makers of this silent crisis. While in developed countries like the USA, the American College of Radiology and other organizations serve as important advocates with Congress or federal agencies or state legislative/regulatory bodies, much remains to be done on this in LMIC. Similar advocacy partners are needed for LMIC in global radiation oncology [14].

Advocacy for greater investment in radiotherapy infrastructure is also needed. WHO and the IAEA have the opportunity to use their leadership roles to mobilize stakeholders into committing to more investment in radiation therapy services. The *Lancet* Oncology Commission report encouraged WHO in particular to engage in a dialogue about cancer treatment and include radiation therapy, which has not typically been part of the discourse. Other national and supranational organizations like the International Agency for Research on Cancer, and the Union for International Cancer Control could also support such dialogue and the need for greater investment in radiotherapy. Multilateral development agencies, civil society professional associations and the private sector are also encouraged to include cancer control and global radiation oncology in their development agendas.

Public–private partnerships

In talking about the private sector and partnerships for global health, public–private partnerships for greater investment in sustainable cancer control programming are highly recommended. Public–private partnerships could strengthen global radiation oncology and supply some of the resources that are desperately needed to support this work. One example is that of the Elekta–Radiating Hope partnership [15]. A number of informed grassroots movements in favor of global radiation oncology are also emerging, for example Global RT [16], a movement led by radiation oncology residents. Diaspora grassroots movements could also be engaged to support cancer prevention education and advocacy campaigns in LMIC, and treatment modalities such as radiotherapy. In addition to promoting cancer education/awareness, it is important to change the perception that oncology is a specialty for pain and death and that radiotherapy is not feasible in LMIC [17].

Align aid with country-led cancer control plans

LMIC typically receive aid from multiple global agencies, which may result in overburdened health ministries. With the majority of investments now being delivered and managed via local nongovernmental organizations operating outside the recipient government's budgeting system, many LMIC struggle to maintain control of their own health priorities. LMIC with weak control of their health systems lose the incentive and ability to create and support their own sustainable plans. To ensure that LMIC retain ownership and accountability for the health of their populations and to promote long-term sustainability, aid should help recipient LMIC in developing results-focused, country-led agreements that rally all development partners around one country-led cancer control plan, where appropriate. In addition, a lack of coordination or synergy with existing national plans may utilize resources inefficiently as efforts are duplicated. This may significantly foster corruption. Where appropriate, it may be useful not to have external funding sources or agencies establish new coordination structures, work outside of the existing health systems, or limit the authority or participation of the existing leadership.

Furthermore, funding sources or agencies should develop new approaches for synergies so that the scarce resources in LMIC are not drained. In one instance, medical physicists from many LMIC countries were sponsored to attend an international conference for a week. However, most of these medical physicists were the only ones available in their LMIC. Although the conference was important, what that meant was that no other medical physicists were available in their respective countries during the week that they were at the conference. This meant that patients suffered. It is for such reasons that funding sources and agencies have often been criticized for weakening existing health systems, because they can lead to internal 'brain drain'.

As said previously, international collaborations need local and transparent leadership, where equitable relationships flourish and ideas are not simply imposed from outside. To achieve this, governments, research institutions and others must work to build a conducive atmosphere of collaborative partnership as a means of working together to achieve a good that is greater than any one agency or enterprise could otherwise achieve on its own. Collaborations such as those modeled as twinning partnerships can improve transparency and streamline efforts with other donors by involving in-country government leadership where appropriate, improving program sustainability and effectiveness.

Universal health coverage

While investment in the development of lower-cost technologies and similar is necessary, there is also a need for increased research and evaluation efforts directed at addressing the systemic bottlenecks in health systems in LMIC that keep the full benefits of existing medical and public health knowledge and technologies from being completely realized. universal health coverage should be seriously considered in LMIC to facilitate access to cancer treatment. Most LMIC citizens have to pay a large portion of their healthcare costs without the benefit of social safety nets. Innovative approaches for universal health coverage should be encouraged.

Accreditation of online education programs

At the 2015 AORTIC conference in Marrakech, it was recommended that the organization take a leading role in accrediting the online education programs in oncology offered for Africans. As more global radiation oncology online education programs become available, having such appropriate organizations in Africa and other continents and regions to provide accreditation services could facilitate their establishment.

Creating medical physicists positions in health ministries in LMIC

Medical physicists play a crucial role in modern medicine. Every hospital or clinic that uses radiation needs qualified medical physicists to ensure that imaging and treatment services are delivered safely and to the highest standards. Table 6.2 shows

Table 6.2. Table showing low compliance in radiation safety in Cameroon for radiation technologies. Data courtesy of Samba Richard.

Type of equipment	Compliance	Acceptable	Non-compliance	Total	% Compliance
Conventional radiology	16	15	19	50	32
Mammography	2	5	0	7	40
Dark room	2	7	14	23	8
View boxes	43	3	23	69	62
Dental radiography	5	0	8	13	38
Total	68	30	64	162	38

an example of the level of compliance in radiation safety control in an LMIC (38%). This is an average for different imaging technologies. The situation is also alarming for radiation technologies for treatment. The expertise of medical physicists and the technologies they develop help to make sure that patients are diagnosed (imaged) and treated correctly in order to survive major illnesses, including cancer, cardiovascular diseases (coronary heart disease, stroke), infectious diseases, appendicitis, trauma, musculoskeletal disorders, and so forth.

A recent survey conducted by the IAEA showed that there is a drastic shortage of qualified medical physicists in hospitals, clinics and health ministries in LMIC in Africa. This drastic shortage is partly due to little or no awareness of the essential role medical physicists have for the benefit of patients (citizens). It is now well recognized that the shortage of qualified medical physicists is a serious problem that requires urgent attention [18–20]. With the alarming increase in the burden of cancer in LMIC in Africa and elsewhere, there is an increasing need for the services of medical physicists. With this in mind, we make the following recommendations.

1. **Medical physicist recognition.** In many LMIC, physicians, e.g. radiation or clinical oncologists, are recognized as health care professionals at the governmental or ministerial level. It is recommended that medical physicists also be recognized as health professionals with specialist education and training in the concepts and techniques of applying physics in medicine, competent to practice independently in one or more of the subfields of medical physics. This is particularly urgent in view of the accounts from Europe and the USA [13] concerning overexposure to radiation resulting from radiological accidents during medical imaging. There are most likely such incidents in Africa that are not being reported. The medical physicists should be involved in:
    i. evaluating each type of practice that has to do with medical exposure, involving the standardization of procedures and the optimization of protection by managing the parameters affecting the dose; each exposure should be evaluated in terms of benefits and risks;
    ii. the calibration and monitoring of imaging equipment to ensure accurate doses are safely delivered to the patients;

iii. organizing and implementing appropriate quality assurance programs, including quality control measures;
iv. assessing radiation doses and associated risks to patients and personnel, especially for pregnant women and children;
v. providing radiation protection education and training to other health professionals, which, together with team working and effective communication, are key components of a safety culture program;
vi. advise on installation design, technical specifications and participate in the procurement, acceptance and commissioning of medical imaging equipment.

As a complement to the recognition of medical physicists, it is recommended that LMIC establish mechanisms so that all centers employing radiation technologies in the country should have access to medical physics services. The LMIC should also recognize that only qualified medical physicists are professionally competent to provide advice on all radiation dose issues, guarantee that all radiological practices comply with national regulations and international guidelines and standards, and ensure that accurate quality control procedures are performed and evaluated on all equipment employing radiation. Furthermore, LMIC should review and enforce legislative and regulatory requirements related to radiation safety, in accordance with the international basic safety standards.

2. **Medical physicist employment.** In many LMIC, medical physicist positions do not exist in the health service structure. It is therefore recommended that LMIC establish posts and employ medical physicists to serve in centers using radiation technologies. LMIC should also put in place appropriate strategies for the retention of clinically qualified medical physicists in health sector career development.
3. **Increased training of medical physicists.** Given the shortage of human capacity in many LMIC, it will be necessary to train more medical physicists to complement the action from the other recommendations. The IAEA, the African Regional Cooperative Agreement on Research, Development and Training related to Nuclear Science and Technology (AFRA), the Federation of African Medical Physics Organisations (FAMPO) and the International Organization for Medical Physicists (IOMP) have been working to harmonize a curriculum for medical physics training. LMIC are encouraged to assess their national training needs related to medical physics and consider the introduction of academic and clinical training programmes, where necessary and justified, based on the minimum requirements presented in the harmonized curriculum developed by AFRA. The LMIC should also develop clear policies for the evaluation of clinical training and subsequent recognition of clinically qualified medical physicists. It is also important to establish a mechanism for the official accreditation or registration of medical physicists by relevant authorities to ensure that minimum training requirements are met. Another recommendation would be for LMIC to promote the regional

harmonization of training programs and mutual recognition of clinically qualified medical physicists to promote the mobility of expertise within the region and facilitate regional equity in care.

Apps for cancer education and awareness and downstaging of cancer
Given that a recent study by Ngoma *et al* showed how education that includes the use of ICTs can significantly downstage cancer, more such ICT-based cancer education and awareness initiatives (e.g. using mobile phone apps) could help downstage cancer and increase the chances of a cure with radiotherapy rather than palliative care. Such cancer education and awareness could also help to demystify radiotherapy and improve cancer prevention awareness/education.

Other recommendations
In an interview with *Global Oncology* [21] Professor Arno Mundt, Chair of the Department of Radiation Medicine and Applied Sciences at the University of California, San Diego, recommended the development of more hypofractionated external beam radiotherapy treatment for LMIC in order to increase the number of patients who undergo treatment, and as a better use of limited resources/infrastructure. This recommendation is somewhat consistent with the TiDTaC technology highlighted in the previous chapter. Another recommendation from Professor Mundt to those looking to become involved in global radiation oncology was that they should not engage in it simply as 'medical tourists'. Longer-term commitment is helpful in gaining the trust and buy-in of physicians and other health professionals on-site in LMIC. Professor Mundt also echoed the need for increased training to ensure sustainability and expressed the hope that radiation oncology professional organizations and vendors will help support the training of more radiation oncologists and physicists throughout the developing world in the coming years.

In another global oncology interview [22], Dr Surbhi Grover, an emerging global radiation oncology leader, also had some advice or recommendations for residents: 'Be curious and passionate—take advantage of the opportunities that come your way even if they don't always seem to fit with the traditional path; be patient, as the best projects and most stimulating ventures take the longest to yield any tangible results.'

At the 2015 Global Health Catalyst summit, global health leaders were asked about what they would recommend based on their experience in collaborating or working with partners in LMIC. Some of the recommendations included the following.

- There should be an equal partnership with high functioning organizations in the LMIC.
- Cultural differences should be respected and taken into account.
- Keep ICT implementation simple.
- Make a significant investment in local capacity.
- Encourage at least short duration site (exchange) visits by collaboration partners.
- Be flexible and ensure regular communication.
- Engage with the LMIC community, build local contacts, build a network, work together.
- Establish trusting human relationships.
- Focus on how to create a sustainable model with education and training at the core.

There are definitely more recommendations that can be made in addition to those featured in this chapter. The ones made here provide a starting point, a useful reference for those looking to engage in this field, and could help shape expectations and goals to maximize impact and foster a positive global health experience.

References

[1] Funding sources www.fic.nih.gov/Funding/NonNIH/Pages/default.aspx

[2] CUGH www.cugh.org/about/mission

[3] In Swaziland, US preacher sees his dream vanish www.wsj.com/articles/SB113495910699726095

[4] Wilkinson's dream for Africa is shattered www.lighthousetrailsresearch.com/dream.pdf

[5] www.wsj.com/articles/SB113495910699726095 Accessed 3 January 2016

[6] Cohen J 2000 Balancing the collaboration equation *Science* **288** 2155–9

[7] Fried L P, Bentley M E, Buekens P, Burke D S, Frenk J J, Klag M J and Spencer H C 2010 Global health is public health *Lancet* **375** 535–7

[8] www.africaneconomicoutlook.org/fileadmin/uploads/aeo/2015/PDF_Chapters/Overview_AEO2015_EN-web.pdf Accessed 3 January 2016

[9] Olson A C, Coleman C N, Hahn S M, DeWeese T L, Shulman L N, Chabner B A, Chao N, Martei Y M, Mundt A J and Grover S 2015 A roadmap for a new academic pathway for global radiation oncology *Int. J. Radiat. Oncol. Biol. Phys.* **93** 493–6

[10] Coleman C N 2014 The international cancer expert corps: a unique approach for sustainable cancer care in low and lower-middle income countries *Front. Oncol.* **4** 333

[11] *Global Health Delivery* www.globalhealthdelivery.org

[12] Report on regional workshop to raise awareness on medical physicists' roles in ensuring safety in imaging—with emphasis on pediatric imaging (Dar es Salaam, Republic of Tanzania, 26–28 November 2014) www.wfpiweb.org/Portals/7/Child%20imaging%20Safety/Dar_WHO_Regional_workshop_report.pdf

[13] Walt B 2010 As technology surges, radiation safeguards lag www.nytimes.com/2010/01/27/us/27radiation.html?hpw

[14] Porter A, Aref A, Chodounsky Z, Elzawawy A, Manatrakul N, Ngoma T, Orton C, Van't Hooft E and Sikora K 1999 A global strategy for radiotherapy: a WHO consultation *Clin. Oncol. (R. Coll. Radiol.)* **11** 368–70

[15] Elekta helps raise $33,000 to bring radiation treatment to developing countries www.elekta.com/press/f76d4e06-f6d3-4e90-b8f4-19fa300b058c/elekta-helps-raise-33-000-to-bring-radiation-treatment-to-developing-countries.html

[16] Rodin D, Yap M L and Hanna T P 2014 GlobalRT: building a new radiotherapy community *Lancet Oncol.* **15** 926

[17] Ngwa W *et al* 2016 *Closing the Cancer Divide through Ubuntu: Information and Communication Technology Powered Models for Global Radiation Oncology* at press

[18] Dendy P and Ringertz H 2002 Serious deficiencies in numbers of medical physics experts in diagnostic radiology *Eur. Radiol.* **12** 2125–6

[19] Thomadsen B 2004 The shortage of radiotherapy physicists *J. Am. Coll. Radiol.* **1** 280–2

[20] Perkins J D 2007 Early development of nanoprobes for diagnostic imaging *Liver Transpl.* **13** 1604

[21] An interview with Dr Arno Mundt—radiation oncology in Africa: improving access to cancer care on the African continent http://globalonc.org/an-interview-with-Dr-arno-mundt-radiation-oncology-in-africa-improving-access-to-cancer-care-on-the-african-continent/

[22] An interview with Dr Surbhi Grover: radiation oncology and global health http://globalonc.org/go-interview-Dr-surbhi-grover/

Chapter 7

Global radiation oncology: *quo vadis*?

The time has come to agree and implement immediate actions to tackle the global shortfall in radiotherapy services and the crisis of access to this highly effective treatment

Rifat Atun, Lancet Oncology Commission [1]

The Lancet Oncology Commission [1] presented a compelling case for greater investment in radiotherapy, showing that this will not only save millions of lives and prevent needless suffering for millions more, but also enable substantial economic returns on investments. The Commission's report concluded by calling for six key targets to be met.

By 2020

- 80% of countries should have comprehensive cancer plans that include radiotherapy.
- Each LMIC should create one new center for treatment and training.
- 80% of LMIC to include radiotherapy services in their universal health coverage plans.

By 2025

- A 25% increase in radiotherapy treatment capacity.
- LMIC to train 7500 radiation oncologists, 20 000 radiotherapy radiographers and 6000 medical physicists.
- 46 billion US dollars of upfront investment to be raised to establish radiotherapy infrastructure and training in LMIC (with help from international banks and the private sector).

Greater global radiation oncology activity or collaborations will be key to meeting these targets. At the recent Global Health Catalyst summit, participants expressed an interest in participating in the following ways: mentorship; education and training, including in online learning; research, including e-research; consulting,

doi:10.1088/978-0-7503-1224-0ch7

including remote consultation; provision of equipment; participation in research and development, e.g. for lower-cost technologies for LMIC; quality assurance support, implementation science; community engagement research; health outcomes research; advice on better value cancer care; grant development; facilitating connections between potential mentors and mentees; facilitating ICT transfers to LMIC; maximizing lifetime value of radiation technologies for customers in LMIC; advocacy; and cancer awareness education. These areas of collaboration and others can be classified into cancer care, research, education and outreach. They are expected to see growth in the future in order for success and the needed progress to be realized.

Cancer care

Many countries will undoubtedly establish new cancer centers with radiotherapy services. LMIC present major opportunities and new markets for greater investment in this. Major radiation technology companies have expressed an interest in making radiotherapy machines and technologies more affordable. It is conceivable that each LMIC will be able to establish at least one new cancer center with radiotherapy services by 2020. Comprehensive cancer centers in developed countries as well as institutions should look to partner more with these centers, including through telemedicine, as highlighted in previous chapters.

ICTs will also increasingly become a major component of clinical care. Remote consultations, tumor boards, treatment planning and quality assurance are expected to see a major increase in activity. The examples or models highlighted in previous chapters will serve as useful references for anyone interested in or planning to begin such activities.

Cancer research

More research collaborations are imperative for the future of global radiation oncology, including for the research and development of lower-cost technologies. There is now talk of making LINACs more like cobalt machines, or making cobalt machines more like LINACs. The development of other approaches or technologies for more affordable radiotherapy, as highlighted in chapter 5, will likely increase, e.g. for technologies that can boost hypofractionation, dramatically cut down treatment times and enable lower-cost access and greater therapeutic efficacy. Greater investment in global radiation oncology research will likely enable the development of more alternative bottom-up technologies in areas like these, which can then also be used in developed countries.

In the years ahead, it is expected that there will be more opportunities for research collaborations between developed country and LMIC partners, including e-research and the use of ICTs to support existing and new forms of research. Such an increase in research will complement educational efforts, e.g. via master's degree or doctoral research projects.

Education and training

A major increase in education and training programs is expected in the coming years, including online education. Each of the new cancer centers established can also partner with developed country institutions in education and training to overcome the dearth of human capacity and expand radiotherapy services. In these efforts new curriculums and international credentialing and accreditation will be required and instituted. The Lancet Oncology Commission proposed a goal of training 7500 radiation oncologists, 20 000 radiation technologists and 6000 medical physicists in LMIC by 2025.

It is also expected that there will be more cancer awareness education, which could help to destigmatize cancer, change the prevailing adverse perceptions about radiotherapy and motivate more people to train in oncology. This is crucial because a cancer diagnosis in many LMIC often spells gloom and sends patients and their caregivers into depression. The fear of side-effects and the cost of cancer treatments also drives many to try alternative therapies. As people become more aware that cancer can be cured if diagnosed early and treated properly, the benefits of such education and awareness can advance global oncology greatly.

Developed-world professional societies like ASTRO and AAPM are likely to increase their collaboration with professional organizations in LMIC, e.g. AORTIC, in education and training efforts. Jakob Van Dyk has put together a comprehensive document on radiation oncology medical physics resources for working, teaching, and learning that could be highly beneficial for global radiation oncology education and training efforts [3].

Outreach

There will clearly be greater outreach to partner and synergize with other global oncology areas such as cancer prevention, surgery and medical oncology. Major partnerships with industry are also envisioned to grow in number and substance. Outreach engagement of community partners is also a potent area for further development.

One group that is expected to play a major role is diaspora communities. This approach is being actively pushed by the Global Health Catalyst program in Harvard and their partners, such as the Harvard African Studies Center and AORTIC. At the recent global health summit, many areas were identified where the diaspora can play a more active role, including the provision of expertise (turning the brain drain into gain against cancer); greater advocacy; cancer education and awareness, which could also benefit their diaspora communities; support for capacity building; serving as global health catalysts because of their multicultural background; helping cut red-tape in LMIC; and supporting universal health coverage in their original LMIC. The support of the diaspora could also facilitate the inclusion of radiotherapy services as part of universal health coverage in many LMIC.

It is also expected that more funding will become available. Until now, the USA and other wealthy nations have mostly invested in infectious diseases like HIV/AIDs. There have also been many public–private partnerships and university-based collaborative research models devoted to global health in the infectious disease arena. One is likely to see more of these in the area of cancer in future.

ICTs are the future
ICTs are the future. They provide powerful tools to facilitate global radiation oncology, e.g. in telemedicine, online education and e-research. Global health leaders expect increased partnerships with ICT companies like Apple, Google, IBM, Microsoft, Samsung, etc, beyond the support from the radiotherapy industry and foundations.

Building on ICTs, LMIC will likely create electronic records for their populations in the future. Many LMIC will likely be able to improve infrastructure faster than high-income countries because of their ability to 'leap frog' onto new technology platforms without transferring from paper records and old ways of doing things. People in LMIC could even take the lead on mobile health, electronic registries and technological innovation.

Conclusion

The rising global burden of cancer and the disparities, including in the provision of radiation oncology services, is alarming. However, the future is hopeful. One of the reasons for hope is the lessons learned from HIV/AIDS. It all seemed impossible and understandably so in the early 2000s. But through concerted efforts and collaborations, remarkable progress has been achieved.

The recognition in 2011 by the United Nations of the growing burden of noncommunicable diseases like cancer in LMIC was a significant step in a hopeful direction [2]. Through concerted action, and with global radiation oncology as a crucial component, major progress towards realizing the vision of eliminating cancer disparities can be made.

Many years ago, the US president John F Kennedy stood before a joint session of the US Congress and said, 'I believe we should go to the Moon'. It was a call to mankind that inspired a generation of Americans in pursuit of science and innovation, where they literally pushed the boundaries of what was possible. With the recent announcement of the 'moonshot to cure cancer' by US president Barack Obama, also before a joint session of Congress, there is hope and excitement in the oncology community. The US government followed this announcement with a two-point execution plan: first for increased resources, both private and public, to support cancer work, and second, for the breaking down of silos and the catalyzation of collaborations and the sharing of information to 'end cancer as we know it'. Altogether, the plan boils down to more resources and collaborations, along with political will, at the highest levels. This execution plan is also relevant in advancing global radiation oncology towards improved healthcare outcomes, millions of saved lives and the elimination of global cancer disparities.

References

[1] Atun R *et al* 2015 Expanding global access to radiotherapy *Lancet Oncol.* **16** 1153–86

[2] United Nations High-level meeting on non-communicable diseases www.un.org/en/ga/president/65/issues/ncdiseases.shtml Accessed 5 January 2016

[3] Van Dyk J (ed) 1999 *The Modern Technology of Radiation Oncology: a Compendium for Medical Physicists and Radiation Oncologists* (Madison, WI: Medical Physics Publishing)

Lightning Source UK Ltd.
Milton Keynes UK
UKOW07n0159060517
300580UK00004B/46/P

9 780750 312257